Cooking

for the

New Hippocratic Diet®

Irving A. Cohen, M.D., M.P.H.

Center for Health Information
Topeka, Kansas
www.centerforhealthinformation.com

Published by
Center for Health Information, Inc.
Suite 22F
1919 SW 10th Avenue
Topeka, KS 66604
Phone (888) 933-9833
FAX (866) 516-1321
e-mail comments@hippocraticdiet.com

Library of Congress Control Number: 2010902851

Cohen, Irving A. 1944-

Cooking for the
New Hippocratic Diet®

ISBN 978-0-9820111-7-1

Editor, Alice Heiserman
Cover Illustrator, Darlene Powell

Printed in the United States of America

Contents

Main Courses - *continued*

Chapter 6. Treats 117

Chapter 7. Condiments 133

This book is dedicated to my family, who has assisted in the development of this collection. In particular, to my wife Lauren, who has patiently developed many of these recipes and tried all of them.

I would like to acknowledge the many dieters, who have suggested, submitted, and shared their recipes and ideas. Recipes and suggestions passed through many hands and underwent many variations, so it became impossible to solely attribute any recipe to a single individual.

Thank you to you all. I hope that this diversity has made the New Hippocratic Diet® more interesting and appealing to a range of people.

Warnings and Disclaimers

- Recipes and food choices discussed in this book
  are intended for those following a special plan.
  These may or may not be the best choices for
  others.

- The information presented in this book has been
  obtained from sources believed to be authentic
  and reliable. Although great care has been taken
  to ensure the accuracy of the information
  presented, the author and the publisher cannot
  assume responsibility for the validity of all the
  materials or the consequences for their use.

- This is a cookbook. Nothing in this book should
  be construed as individual medical advice. Any
  reader needing such personal advice should
  consult his or her own physician.

1

Basic Information

Welcome to *Cooking for the New Hippocratic Diet®* . Before skipping to the recipes, take the time to learn the purpose of and some of the conventions used in this book. Are you familiar with the New Hippocratic Diet®? This book is intended for those following this plan and for others who may be cooking for them. The New Hippocratic Diet® is aimed at two audiences and is described in a series of books.

The first group is made up of people who are overweight and have been unable to succeed in losing weight using more conventional plans. Today, that means about two out of three American adults. *Dr. Cohen's New Hippocratic Diet® Guide: How to Really Lose Weight and Beat the Obesity Epidemic (ISBN 978-0-9820111-9-5)* explains how this plan works for those needing to lose weight. It works particularly well for those who must lose large amounts of weight to improve their health.

The second group consists of type 2 diabetics. This plan will help some diabetics reduce or eliminate their need for diabetic medication, yet achieve better control than was possible while taking medication. This, in turn, will help prevent the many medical consequences of type 2 diabetes, such as heart disease, kidney failure, blindness, and neuropathy. *Diabetes Recovery: Reversing Diabetes with the New Hippocratic Diet®* *(ISBN 978-0-9820111-0-2)* is intended for them.

If you are in either these categories, I hope you have turned to one of these books. This plan is much more than just a collection of recipes. If you're following this plan for yourself, you'll need to understand the principles involved and not merely look up recipes. Both of these books contain a few starter recipes and the purpose of this book is to provide additional recipes.

Many of these recipes came from my patients. Once they understood the principles of this dietary plan, they scoured cookbooks, the Internet, and their own imagination and creativity to develop new recipes that met the strict criteria of following either of these plans.

Experienced dieters will tell you most diets are a drudgery, while dieters who succeed at the New Hippocratic Diet® describe it as eye-opening and enjoyable. Over the past three decades, Americans have been exposed to significant misinformation about nutrition. Some of this is due to profit-making motives of major food processing companies, but some of the blame belongs to the federal government.

While trying to make all Americans healthier, the government began giving out incorrect dietary advice three decades ago. This has led to a quadrupling of the number of American adults considered overweight or obese!

The reasons are explained in either of the two books mentioned. The purpose of this book is to give people following the plan additional ideas, varieties, and choices. Readers outside the United States will find measurement conversion information in Appendix A.

Recipes in this book may or may not be appropriate for others. If you need a general description of the plan, you might call it a very low carbohydrate, moderate protein and moderate fat plan. People following the plan are monitoring the amount of these nutrients that they are eating.

In many ways, it is totally the opposite of the largely discredited food pyramid that many Americans still think is "healthy eating". If that food pyramid were healthy, then why do those who follow it end up helplessly overweight and diabetic? Visit a cattle producing region to see the answer. The pyramid that the government suggested to lose weight is used by cattle producers to fatten their cattle.

Generally, the recipes in this book are safe and appropriate for everyone, when eaten in the portion size suggested. However, they can not be recommended for people who will eat larger portions than suggested here or who will eat them along with large amounts of sugar.

Each recipe contains nutritional information for a single serving. These nutritional amounts have been calculated multiple ways. In looking at the nutritional content of individual ingredients, standard preferences and manufacturer's product information were used, but were not always accurate. As an example, in the

Basic Information

United States, food packaging companies are allowed to hide the nutritional impact of certain ingredients by keeping the portion size small enough so that their stated content is under a gram and they round down to zero. This practice is not seen in the European Union, where this nutritional content for ingredients is shown in smaller increments.

Next, there is the problem of varying ingredients. We have usually tried to use generic terms for products. This ignores the small differences between one supplier or another. For instance, did you know that avocados grown in California and Florida are different in their nutritional content? Each state has its own agricultural marketing association, providing different information for what most consumers would think is the same product. Then again, sometimes the avocados you see in a store come from Mexico or another country and even less is known about them.

Another problem arises from using currently available nutritional analysis software. Because such software makes assumptions about the content of ingredients, such analysis can only be considered an estimate. We have used a variety of methods, using both computer estimates and manually calculated estimates.

Next, there are the hidden ingredients. One example is that little packet of "non-calorie" sweetener you may have used in your coffee or tea recently. Read the label. It tells you that it contains zero calories; yet, when you read the ingredient list, the first ingredient is often sugar. The food industry considers this a "flowing agent," something that they use to make this sweetener dissolve the same way as real sugar. Often, this flowing agent is ordinary sugar!

When used in small amounts, such as a single packet, it may be of little consequence. However, many of the same products come in baking and cooking varieties, encouraging you to use a cup or more. Do they tell you that there's a lot of sugar in their product? No, they continue to give the same nutritional misinformation by showing you the nutritional breakdown for a tiny amount, even though the packaging encourages you to use a cup. In some cases, it was necessary to go into scientific analyses of these products to estimate their true nutritional content.

Then there is the government, again. In order to assure fairness , the government requires the use of a century-old technique of "objectively" measuring the caloric content by the amount of heat food generates when burned. This is actually not objective, because people are not furnaces!

This does not take into account foods that will burn, but cannot be digested. For example, cattle can digest grass, but humans can not. The cellulose found in grass is an indigestible fiber, but produces energy when burned. This leads to misleading and confusing information. In this book, we have done the required calculation and only provided energy that actually may be used. In the case of carbohydrates, this is sometimes referred to as "net carbs." In this book, all carbohydrate values given are for such net carbs.

Finally, there are individual differences. How you digest food may depend upon how well you chew or what helpful bacteria live in your gastrointestinal tract. How a food is digested may also depend upon the exact way a particular food is cooked or trimmed. Any nutritional analysis, anywhere, is at best, approximate. Monitor what you eat and how it affects you.

All recipes in this cookbook specify number of servings and portion size. Portion control is essential in both weight-loss dieting and diabetes control. It is a myth that there are "safe foods" that anyone can eat with impunity. People keep looking for these "magic foods" because it seems like an easy path. Nothing could be further from the truth.

Each recipe contains a breakdown of usable macronutrient energy. This is shown in grams of fat, protein, and carbohydrate. During the weight-loss phase, dieters are instructed to have a set amount of each of these daily. For many people, 60 grams of fat, 40 grams of protein, and 10 grams of carbohydrate is a reasonable starting point. This is intended for adults who are not healing from a serious illness. It is not for pregnant women. Once dieters reached their goal weight, they should adjust their diet to keep their weight stable, and provide sufficient energy for daily activity. In the case of diabetics, stable blood sugar control that minimizes the need for medication is the important goal.

The listings for grams of carbohydrate take into account poorly digested forms of carbohydrate and only state net amounts. All meals should roughly balance these proportions, so that each meal is a mixture. Finally, there is nothing sacred about eating three meals a day. People on high carbohydrate plans often graze because they are hungry between meals. This plan has the opposite effect. Many will often find that they are not hungry at traditional mealtimes and adjust the number and frequency of meals that they eat, accordingly. Interestingly, the customary number, size and timing of meals varies in different cultures.

Measurements are stated in ways common in the average kitchen. The term "ounces" is not used in this book for fluid measure, so whenever ounces is used, it means weight, not volume. All the volume measurements are listed in terms of cups and spoons.

Generally, we have avoided brand names. When specific products are called for, it is because they seem to be either unique or clearly superior. We have tried to keep this to minimum, but sometimes there is a wide discrepancy between *Product A* and *Product B*.

Sugar is always avoided. There is absolutely nothing essential about sugar in the diet. Indeed, sugar was once considered one of the "rare spices," and information about sugar processing was kept a state secret in the ancient India and Persia. It was not until the European powers began the mass cultivation of sugar in the Americas using African slaves that the price of sugar began to fall to a point where its use became common. Throughout history, going back to ancient India, whenever sugar usage increased there was a corresponding increase in certain types of disease.

Today, many myths exist regarding "healthy sugar." These myths can be traced to public relations, spin originating from the associations and companies involved in sugar production and sales.

Sugar substitutes always present a dilemma. Again, many myths exist. In general, there are issues with some of the substitutes, but the greatest offender is sugar itself. Either avoid sweeteners entirely or find the ones best suited for you.

Fortunately, today there are a variety of artificial sweeteners, and if you have difficulty with one type, you have a number of choices. Differences exist from one nation to another regarding which of these artificial sweeteners is considered safe. Brand name products often change formulation as borders are crossed.

In the United States, the biggest myth about artificial sweeteners is that they are all calorie-free. Since many use a flowing agent, which is usually a carbohydrate such as sugar, they do have calories. By craftily wording labels, manufacturers are able to legally pretend that these sweeteners have no energy. Usually, this is untrue.

Avoid these flowing agents by using a liquid non-calorie sweetener. Liquid sweeteners do not need to use these flowing agents, instead only using water. A few baked items need the texture of a solid, so occasionally we include granulated sweeteners as an ingredient. Feel free to experiment and replace these wherever possible.

Which sweeteners are best? The two that I suggest everyone try are liquid saccharin and liquid *Stevia*. Although these sweeteners are available in a solid form, using them in their liquid form avoids the carbohydrate-containing flowing agents. One advantage to liquid sweeteners is that you only need a few drops.

Saccharin was the original artificial sweetener and has been in use for over a century. One drawback for saccharin is that some people notice a bitter aftertaste when using it in large amounts. Another issue is the question about safety. Saccharin was falsely accused of being "dangerous" because chemically it was originally derived from coal tar. Coal tar, when continuously applied to the skin, is an irritant that can cause cancer at the location to which it was applied. The chemicals that are derived from coal tar are not inherently dangerous. However, in the 1950's, scientists were able to create skin tumors in rats using saccharin at a strength 100,000 times normal. So far, other than occasional allergic sensitivity, there has not been any association between human disease and saccharin use. However, in the 1970s a new form of artificial sweetener came to the market. This was cyclamate and it quickly became popular. There was intense lobbying to get the government to ban saccharin in the United States, and it almost worked. However, before the government could ban saccharin, laboratory experiments showed that cyclamate, under certain conditions, could harm the kidney. That caused the U.S. government to ban cyclamate and leave saccharin alone. On the other hand, the Canadian government had acted more rapidly and banned saccharin. They have left cyclamate alone, so the same brand name of artificial sweetener in the United States and in Canada actually contain different ingredients. In the United States, liquid saccharin can be found in most supermarkets along with baking ingredients.

Stevia is a newer form of sweetener. It is derived from the leaf of a small plant originating in South America. Some people may be successful in growing this in their home herb garden. Because it is sweet in its natural form, many people consider this a "natural" sweetener. Large food corporations have used it outside the United States to sweeten diet soft drinks. It was delayed in the United States until recently, when an artificially processed form of it was approved. However, before that approval, many companies began to offer it legally as a herbal substitute. In this unaltered form, it may be found in a liquid form at health and nutrition stores.

Aspartame is a popular artificial sweetener that came to the market shortly after cyclamate was banned in the U.S. It is popular because many people think that it is close to the taste of sugar. However, it has serious drawbacks. First of all, it must never be used in cooking. When heated, it may break down into toxic chemicals such as formaldehyde and wood alcohol. Secondly, in liquid form, such as in soft drinks, it should be stored at a cool temperature and used rather rapidly. This was not widely recognized in until the 1990s when U.S. forces in the middle-eastern desert were sent diet soft drinks that were stored in hot warehouses. Since that time, soft drink manufacturers have put a freshness date on their diet products. Pay attention to that date. Although we allow soft drinks on this plan, we encourage alternatives to the commercially available sweetened drinks. This is discussed in Chapter 5.

Aspartame has another problem. Because it uses a modified form of the amino acid aspartate, scientists fear that it may overload brain chemistry and cause long-lasting harm. Today, some physicians and scientists suspect that substances like this may be excitotoxins, chemicals that overstimulate neurons of your brain and cause disease. The diseases they have hypothesized may be linked to this food additive and similar excitotoxins include autism and ALS. Parkinson's disease is another possibility. None of this is proven yet, but there is enough in these arguments to use these products with caution.

Acesulfame is another of the newer sweeteners. Some scientists are concerned that it contains methylene chloride, a chemical which may induce cancers.

Sucralose is a newer sweetener that is made by taking sucrose, a common form of sugar, and attaching a chlorine atom to it. In its powdered form, it is touted as an exact replacement for sugar and is used for supposedly low-carbohydrate baking. Although it performs that function admirably, it must be used carefully. The flowing agent mixed with it is the starch maltodextrin, so it has more carbohydrate than people are led to believe. It is used in some recipes in Chapter 6, but use as little as possible.

Finally, there are the *sugar alcohols*. These chemicals are similar to a sugar with extra atoms of oxygen and hydrogen (called an alcohol group) attached. Your taste buds will sense the sugary part, but your gastrointestinal tract cannot digest the sugar because of the extra alcohol group. These sugar alcohols are found in most sugar-free candies, mints, gum, and ice-cream. Used in moderation, most people can tolerate sugar alcohol. Their downside is that the bacteria that live in your gut love them. The more you eat, the more these bacteria grow and produce gas, cramps, and diarrhea. Individual's reaction to sugar alcohol will vary, since individual's gastrointestinal bacteria varies. The names of most sugar alcohols end in the letters "OL", so you can tell if something is a sugar alcohol. To avoid overuse, it is best to not include these products in sugar-free treats you make yourself.

Another group of substances that must be avoided are the flavor enhancers. These turn common amino acids into drugs that interfere with our normal processing of taste. The most common of these is monosodium glutamate or MSG, a chemical rarely found in nature. It tricks the part of our nervous system associated with taste into believing that artificially flavored foods have a wonderful taste. Despite the spin coming from the food additive manufacturers, this is not a natural event.

Glutamate is a natural amino acid found in the protein that we eat and used by your brain in very important pathways. MSG interferes with the natural glutamate pathways in our bodies. Many people have an unusual reactions to excessive amounts of this chemical. MSG is also suspected of causing neurological disease. Nevertheless, the food lobby has kept it legal through a variety of means. As processed foods have become more and more artificial, this chemical has increased in our food supply to incredible levels.

This increase is one of the underlying causes of our current obesity epidemic. It was proven almost half a century ago that if you add MSG to the food supply of laboratory animals they will eat more and get fat. Enough said.

In the United States, the problem avoiding foods with MSG is that manufacturers know that some consumers are wary of this product. Therefore, they go to great lengths to hide it. Again, they have influenced regulations to suit their needs. By putting MSG into products in an impure form, they only list the materials used to create this drug rather than calling it what it is. Recently, they have gotten so daring that they advertise foods as being "free" of MSG with a small and confusing footnote, which states just the opposite.

There are many names that are used to hide MSG. The industry refers to it as *HVP* or *hydrolyzed vegetable protein*. Ingredient labels will sometimes call it *vegetable protein, soy protein, vegetable broth, yeast extract* and many other similar names. Products labeled for use in the European Union follow a different convention and may have a code between E600 and E699 on their label.

All of these forms of MSG should be avoided totally. Because MSG is actually a drug that fools our nervous system into making bland foods tasty, it triggers a response to eat more. This is sabotage for the dieter.

Are there other reasons to avoid flavor enhancers? Yes, these chemicals are believed to be excitotoxins, as described earlier. However, the person following either a diet to lose weight or a plan to control diabetes can avoid the scientific controversy altogether. The plain facts are that these chemicals make people eat more than they intend to. That should be enough to stop anyone reading this book from using flavor enhancers.

Spices are fine. Real spices, properly used, enhance cooking. Spice mixtures, however, should be viewed with suspicion. Although there are many excellent spice mixtures on the market, be sure to read the ingredient list completely. A significant number of spice mixtures include MSG in one of its forms. Avoid bottled sauces, since many contain both sugar and MSG. Make your own instead. Do not use packaged soups or soup mixes as a flavoring ingredient for any dish. They generally contain highly concentrated MSG.

Do not be afraid to use healthy oil. Consider extra-virgin olive oil as the best all-around oil. Unrefined sesame oil is a wonderful light oil for use on salads. Peanut oil may be considered for high-temperature cooking. Do not be afraid of using butter but avoid all forms of margarine and shortening. Salted butter is preferred, because "unsalted" butter often contains chemical additives.

Store a stick of butter at room temperature. This can be done without the butter going bad by using a special butter keeper. These are found in kitchen supply stores and use a water seal to keep air from reaching your butter. Properly served at room temperature, a pat of butter can easily to added to dishes at your table.

Consider using unrefined coconut oil if you have problems digesting other fats and oils. That is particularly true for people who have been unfortunate enough to have had gallbladder disease and had their gallbladder surgically removed.

Whenever mayonnaise is called, for use real mayonnaise. *Real mayonnaise* is a legal definition requiring the use of oil and egg yolk. Avoid light mayonnaise and mayonnaise substitutes. Whenever cream is called for, use heavy whipping cream. If possible, avoid the ultrapasteurized creams which often contain extra additives. Fresh cream is always preferred. Whenever sour cream is called for, use natural sour cream. Never use light or fat-free products.

Many people attempt to eat healthy foods by buying organic or natural produce. Although their intent is good, the large food companies have twisted the meaning so people are spending money without necessarily getting the benefit they think they are. These products are best if gotten directly from the small farmer or grown in your own backyard. Although there are standards for use of the term "organic," that does not stop the food processors from modifying these products with unhealthy chemicals after they are harvested.

The government allowed use of the term "natural" is so strange that it defies belief. Under U.S. regulations, natural means anything that grows in nature. One example is the strawberry color found in certain "strawberry" dairy products. The label reads *natural food coloring*, which leaves consumers to assume the coloring comes from strawberries. It actually is a red dye that comes from crushed beetles! This one ingredient has been subject to legal attack for many years and the government has finally decided to require food processors to call this *"carmine" color* instead of natural color. What a small victory! There are literally hundreds of other such products where the consumer is being fooled. Since it took over a decade to get the regulation changed for just this one additive, until there is a major shift in government regulation, the word natural never means what people think it means.

There is no restriction on salt use in this plan. Of course, if you have any condition that requires you to restrict your salt use, continue to follow it. Potassium chloride, found in common "salt substitutes", helps maintain a healthy balance between sodium and potassium, two important minerals. What about all those news headlines that Americans must restrict their use of table salt? They are usually misquoting scientific recommendations that Americans reduce their **sodium** intake. Table salt (sodium chloride) contains sodium, but so does **monosodium** glutamate and other variations of flavor-enhancing drugs. It is the addition of these additives that is responsible for the sodium imbalance in the processed foods. By avoiding these flavor enhancers, you have already reduced your sodium intake!

All of this may sound complicated and mystifying, if you are not already following this plan. It is not, for once you make the switch to real food, you will find it both tastier and healthier.

Appendix B shows you how to calculate the nutritional analysis for a serving of your own recipes. If you have recipes you would like to share, send them by e-mail to *comments@HippocraticDiet.com*.

Appendix C shows you how to record and monitor your progress on this plan.

2

Main Courses

What does it take to be a main course? Included in this chapter are dishes that some people would consider main courses but to others they might seem like appetizers. Have you ever ordered a platter of mixed appetizers at an Asian restaurant or gone to a Spanish-style *tapas* bar, which serves small portions of a variety of tasty dishes? Those small appetizers can also become a main course.

This chapter is broken down into sections by the type of main course, but your choice of main courses can be as varied as your experience, background, and imagination leads you to be. Do not get too hung up differentiating between what should be an appetizer and what should be a main course. If it works, and meets the basic outline of this plan, do it and enjoy it.

Main Courses

Beef.

Beef is the quintessential American main course. In this section, we are not giving you instructions on basics, such as classic burgers or steaks, but they are fine! The recipes here give you some extra ways to dress up these traditional dishes.

Be very careful when purchasing meats. Avoid portion-controlled frozen steaks, which are often loaded with chemicals. Many of today's supermarket chains sell meat that has been pre-packaged at a distant slaughtering plant. The people behind the counter wearing white butcher coats may know nothing about meat cutting and butchering. Instead, they simply take pre-cut meat from packages and put it in the display case. The danger here is that this meat is likely to be injected with flavor-enhancing chemicals.

The word *natural* on the packaging provides little to guide you in this regard. If you are lucky, you may be able to buy meats from animals raised at a small farm and processed at a country butcher or locker plant. These choices are fast disappearing, since the federal government has burdened these small businesses with regulations designed for massive assembly-line plants.

Remember that natural saturated fat, in moderate quantity, is normal. The old-fashioned standards of marbled meat with some fat left on produce the tastiest meats and, if they contain more fat than you wish to eat, they can be trimmed after they have been cooked.

Grilled Citrus Steak
Serves 4

Ingredient	Amount
Top sirloin steak	1 pound
Olive oil	½ cup
Kosher or sea salt	To taste
Black pepper	To taste
Chopped parsley	¼ cup
Chopped oregano	½ tablespoon
Minced garlic	½ clove
Chili pepper flakes	½ dash
Minced onion	½ tablespoon
Lemon juice	½ tablespoon
Lime juice	½ tablespoon
Wine or malt vinegar	½ tablespoon

Instructions: Preheat grill to medium heat. Season steak with 2 tablespoons olive oil and salt and pepper. Cook for approximately 8 to 10 minutes per side, or until meat reaches an internal temperature of 130 degrees F as measured on a meat thermometer for medium-rare doneness. Put remaining ingredients in a blender and pulse to create sauce, but do not puree. Add salt and pepper to taste. When the steak is cooked to your liking, remove it from the grill and let it rest 7 minutes before slicing. Slice meat across the grain into ¼ inch slices. Serve covered with sauce.

Energy	269	calories
Fat	18	grams
Protein	23	grams
Carbohydrates	2	grams

Main Courses

Flank Steak Grilled with Vegetables
Serves 6

Ingredient	Amount
Flank steak	1 pound
Kosher or sea salt	½ tablespoon, to taste
Pepper	½ tablespoon, to taste
Eggplant	1
Bell peppers	2
Olive oil	6 tablespoons
Wine or malt vinegar	2 tablespoons
Chopped garlic	1 clove
Chopped parsley	½ cup

Instructions: Heat grill to medium-high heat. Season the steak with some of the salt and pepper. Grill to desired doneness, 4 to 5 minutes per side for medium-rare. Transfer to cutting board and let steak rest 5 minutes before slicing across the grain. Meanwhile, slice eggplant and peppers. Brush both sides of the eggplant and peppers with half of the oil. Season with remaining salt and pepper. Grill until tender, 4 to 5 minutes per side. In a small bowl combine the remaining oil, vinegar, garlic, and parsley. Divide the steak and vegetables among individual plates. Spoon the sauce over the vegetables or serve on the side.

Energy	287	**calories**
Fat	22	**grams**
Protein	16	**grams**
Carbohydrate	5	**grams**

Mexican Beef

Serves 4

Ingredient	Amount
Ground beef (80/20)	12 ounces.
Chopped onion	⅓ cup
Chopped bell pepper	½ cup
Water	⅔ cup
Chili powder	1 teaspoon
Ground cumin	1 teaspoon
Tomato Juice	1 cup

Instructions: Sauté beef and onion in a skillet with oil, cumin, and chili powder until tender and brown, stirring frequently. Add remaining ingredients. Lower heat and simmer about 30 minutes.

Energy	**344 calories**
Fat	**29 grams**
Protein	**15 grams**
Carbohydrate	**4 grams**

Main Courses

Mexican Steak
Serves 4

Ingredients	Amount
Chuck steak	12 ounces
Olive oil	1 tablespoon
Herdez® picante sauce	7 ounce can
Lime juice	2 tablespoons
Ground pepper	¼ teaspoon
Chopped cilantro	¼ cup

Instructions: Cut steak into 4 portions. Add oil to frying pan and place over medium heat until hot. Add steak, cook 2 minutes on each side. Combine picante, lime juice and pepper and pour over steak. Cover, reduce heat and simmer 10 minutes. Sprinkle with cilantro.

Energy	236	calories
Fat	17	grams
Protein	14	grams
Carbohydrate	6	grams

Mexican Burgers
Serves 2

Ingredient	Amount
Ground beef (80/20)	6 ounces
Chopped onion	1 tablespoon
Chopped bell peppers	⅓ cup
Chopped cilantro	1 tablespoon
Chopped chili pepper	1 tablespoon
Chopped garlic	1 clove
Ground cumin	½ teaspoon

Instructions: Preheat grill. Combine all ingredients in a small bowl, mixing thoroughly. Shape into patties and cook to taste.

Energy	284	calories
Fat	23	grams
Protein	15	grams
Carbohydrate	4	grams

Main Courses

Casseroles

Casseroles give a comfortable, homemade feeling to a meal. These casseroles are different than those that you were used to. Standard casseroles are often loaded with carbohydrates. Those made with soup are often loaded with MSG. Instead, all of these casseroles are made with healthy and delicious ingredients. Try some.

Asparagus Casserole
Serves 6
A great vegetarian main course.

Ingredient	Amount
Butter	3 tablespoons
Asparagus	2 cups
Onion	1 small *(optional)*
Pepper	to taste
Real sour cream	1 cup
Shredded Swiss cheese	1 cup

Instructions: Melt 2 tablespoons butter in skillet. Next, sauté asparagus until barely tender (2 to 4 minutes). Remove asparagus and place in a baking dish. Using the same skillet, add the remaining tablespoon of butter, slice the onion and sauté until soft but not brown. Now, stir in pepper, sour cream and cheese. Cook over low heat until cheese melts. Pour over asparagus in baking dish. Bake in oven at 350^0 F for 20 minutes or until brown.

Energy	221	calories
Fat	19	grams
Protein	8	grams
Carbohydrate	5	grams

Main Courses

Cauliflower and Cheese Bake
Serves 4

Tasty main course.

Ingredients	Amount
Butter	2 tablespoons
Pork rinds (unflavored)	1 cup
Cauliflower	10 ounces
Cheddar cheese (sharp)	4 ounces

Instructions: Allow the butter to soften to room temperature. Cook the cauliflower, then place it in a greased 1 quart casserole dish. Cut the cheese into ½ inch cubes. Place the pork rinds into a plastic bag and crush them. Top the cauliflower with cheese and butter. Sprinkle the pork rind crumbs on top. Cover the casserole and bake in an oven that has been pre-heated to 350^0. Bake about 20 minutes, until cheese is melted.

Energy	243 calories
Fat	19 grams
Protein	15 grams
Carbohydrate	2 grams

Chili Relleño Casserole

Serves 9

Tasty and spicy cheese casserole.

Ingredients	Amount
Low-carb tortillas	3
Pepperjack cheese	4 slices
Shredded Mexican cheese	1¼ cup
Cream	¾ cup
Eggs	3
Green chili peppers, chopped	4 cans, 4½ ounces each
Chopped onion	½ teaspoon
Salt	½ teaspoon, to taste

Instructions: Grease 8 x 8 inch baking pan. Lay first tortilla in bottom of pan. Drain green chili peppers and spread over tortilla. Spread pepperjack slices next, then cover with ½ cup shredded Mexican cheese. Beat eggs, cream, onion, and salt. Spread half this mixture over this layer. Place second tortilla over that mixture, creating another layer. Add remaining chili peppers. Pour remaining egg mixture over this. Top with remaining shredded Mexican cheese. Bake 35 minutes in a 350⁰ oven. Remove from oven and allow to cool at least 10 minutes before cutting into 9 equal servings.

Energy	124	calories
Fat	10	grams
Protein	6	grams
Carbohydrate	4	grams

Lasagna

Serves 12

Try this delicious lasagna made without noodles. Page 59 discusses other ways to make familiar pasta recipes.

<u>Ingredients</u>	<u>Amount</u>	
Ground beef (80/20)	1	pound
Sausage	¼	pound
Onions (chopped)	½	cup
Tomatoes (crushed)	1	cup
Garlic (minced)	2	cloves
Olive oil	4	teaspoons
Thyme	¼	teaspoon
Salt	1 ½	teaspoons
Pepper	½	teaspoon
Oregano	1	teaspoon
Ricotta cheese	2	cups
Eggs	2	
Spinach, chopped	2	cups *or 10 ounces frozen*
Mushrooms (sliced)	2	cups
Monterey Jack cheese	2	cups, shredded
Celery (chopped)	3	stalks

Lasagna *(continued)*

Instructions: Sauté meat in oil, remove to a plate, and sauté onions, celery and spices together. Add garlic when onions are transparent, then add mushrooms and cook until soft. Mix meat back into onion mixture and add the tomatoes and let simmer a few minutes. Spread into bottom of a large baking pan. Sauté spinach and layer on top of the meat mixture. Mix ricotta cheese and egg and then add other cheese, layer on top of spinach, and bake at 350^0 until brown and cheese is melted, 40-50 minutes.

Energy	345	**calories**
Fat	27	**grams**
Protein	19	**grams**
Carbohydrate	4	**grams**

Main Courses

Ricotta Cheese Soufflé
Serves 4

Works well as a vegetarian main course.

Ingredients	**Amount**	
Butter	1	teaspoon
Eggs	4	
Cream of tartar	1	teaspoon
Ricotta cheese	2	cups
Calorie-free liquid sweetener	5-10	drops, to taste

Instructions: Allow butter to soften to room temperature. Preheat the oven to 300^0. Butter a 9-inch round baking pan. Separate the egg whites and yolks. Beat the egg whites until frothy but not stiff. Add the cream of tartar and continue to beat until you can form high peaks. In a medium–sized bowl, combine the ricotta cheese, egg yolks, and sweetener, and mix well. Fold in the egg whites, gently. Pour the mixture into the baking ban and place it in the oven. Bake for 25 to 30 minutes. Change to broil and broil the top for 2 to 3 minutes, but be careful not to burn the soufflé

Energy	298	calories
Fat	22	grams
Protein	20	grams
Carbohydrate	5	grams

Chili

Some people consider chili the ultimate comfort food. Recipes on the next pages provide three variations of this classic dish, all without beans. Combining beef and pork provides a tasty dish, but some people may prefer all one meat. Be careful about prepared spice or flavoring mixes that may contain diet-busting flavor enhancers.

Do not be afraid of making a large batch. If you are not having friends over to share, freeze it in individual portion sizes. It will reheat easily in the microwave.

Some people like to top their chili with either shredded cheese or sour cream.

Main Courses

Chili # 1

Serves 6

This all beef, bean-less chili may be served with unflavored pork rinds or topped with sour cream.

Ingredient	Amount
Ground beef (80/20)	1 ¼ pounds
Green onions	2 small
Garlic (minced)	1 teaspoon
Chili powder	2 tablespoons
Tomato paste	2 tablespoons
Water	1 ½ cup
Salt and ground pepper	2 teaspoons each, to taste
Shredded cheddar cheese	¼ cup

Instructions: Crumble ground beef and brown in a large pan. Add onions and garlic to the pan and sauté at a lower temperature. Add seasonings and tomato paste. Add water and stir until mixture is combined. Bring to a soft boil stirring occasionally. Lower heat to simmer, top with cheese, and allow flavors to mix.

Energy	318	calories
Fat	27	grams
Protein	17	grams
Carbohydrate	1	grams

Chili # 2

Serves 6

This is another simple and quick all-beef chili.

Ingredients	Amount
Ground beef (80/20)	1 pound
Olive oil	2 tablespoons
Onion flakes	2 teaspoons
Chili powder	To taste
V8™ juice	5½ ounces or 1 small can
Water	5½ ounces
Basil	1 teaspoon

Instructions: In a skillet, brown 1 pound ground beef in olive oil. Next, add V8™ juice and water. Add seasoning to taste Simmer on low heat for 15 minutes, serve. You may wish to add cheese or sour cream as a topping, or serve it with pork rinds.

Energy	282	calories
Fat	25	grams
Protein	19	grams
Carbohydrate	2	grams

Chili # 3

Serves 12

This chili takes longer, but it is our favorite.

Ingredient	Amount	
Ground beef (80/20)	1	pound
Pork sausage (*MSG-free*)	1	pound
Olive oil	2	tablespoons
Diced tomatoes with green chilies	10	ounce can
Crushed tomatoes	10	ounce can
Cumin	2	tablespoons
Chili powder	2	tablespoons
Crushed red pepper	1	teaspoon
Salt and pepper		to taste

Instructions: Crumble the beef and pork sausage, adding it to the oil a bit at a time in a hot frying pan or large heavy pot. Use half the cumin while browning the meat, stirring as you add it. If using a frying pan, now transfer contents to a Crock-Pot® or slow cooker. Now, add all remaining ingredients, stirring well. Adjust to a very low heat and cover. Stir occasionally, do not allow it to stick and burn on the bottom. Cook several hours to bring out the full flavor. You may wish to add a bit of sour cream or shredded cheese on top when serving, or provide pork rinds for party dipping.

Energy	301	calories
Fat	28	grams
Protein	11	grams
Carbohydrate	2	grams

Eggs

Eggs, a healthy food choice, have been maligned over the years. At one time, health experts suggested that Americans eat one egg everyday. Eggs are a balanced source of nutrition combining protein, fat, and little carbohydrate. At the start of the cholesterol scare, consumers were wrongly warned of the cholesterol in egg yolks. This was incorrect, since eating cholesterol is not the controlling factor in your body. It is a high sugar diet that causes your body to make too much of the bad form of cholesterol.

Today, there has been a complete turnaround. Eggs can be made to contain healthy omega-3 fatty acids, simply by altering the feed of chickens. These super-healthy eggs are now marketed in every supermarket, with their packaging boasting of their healthy omega-3 content. The healthiest of eggs are probably the barnyard variety. If you know someone that raises a few chickens for their eggs and lets them roam free, you may have been lucky enough to have tasted eggs with very dark, rich yolks.

It is always dangerous to eat raw eggs. Mass-production egg farms are contaminated with salmonella. Never eat undercooked or runny eggs. None of our recipes use eggs without cooking. Avoid undercooked eggs unless you can find sterilized irradiated eggs.

Eggs do not have to be just for breakfast. Main dishes made from eggs work well with any meal. When traveling, hard boiled eggs, kept cool and in their shells, are a handy food.

Do not fear eggs, enjoy them.

Deviled Eggs

Serves 4 (2 halves per serving)

These are a summertime favorite.
Remember to keep refrigerated once made.

Ingredients	*Amount*	
Eggs	4	large
Mayonnaise	2	tablespoons
Liquid sweetener	¼	teaspoon or 12 drops, to taste
Cider vinegar	½	teaspoon
Salt	⅛	teaspoon
Hot Sauce	1 or 2	drops, to taste
Paprika		To taste

Instructions: Boil eggs until hard. Cool, shell, and peel. Slice eggs in half, lengthwise. Put whites on a plate, yolks in a bowl. Smash yolks into a paste. Add all other ingredients except paprika and whip with fork or whisk. Take by teaspoonfuls and divide evenly, filling the egg white shells. Sprinkle paprika over top. Refrigerate until ready to serve. Wrap remainder with plastic wrap to keep until eaten.

Hint: Some folks like to take a bit of cream cheese softened to room temperature and substitute it for part of the mayonnaise.

Energy	129	calories
Fat	11	grams
Protein	6	grams
Carbohydrate	1	grams

Fluffy Egg Omelet

1 serving

Nutritionally, this is the same as an omelet made in the normal way but once you try it, you will appreciate its flavor, texture, and size. Using a single egg, it provides about the same size portion as an ordinary two egg omelet. If you are not used to separating eggs, buy a simple egg separator at a kitchen or housewares store.

Ingredients	*Amount*
Large egg	1
Heavy cream	1 teaspoon
Extra-virgin olive oil (or butter)	1 teaspoon
Salt, pepper, or spice	To taste

Instructions: Separate the egg white from the yolk. Using an electric mixer or a hand whisk, beat the egg white until it is very frothy and increased in volume. Heat the olive oil (or butter) in a frying pan. Lightly blend the egg yolk and spices into the frothy egg white. Pour the mixture into the heated frying pan. Cook until done, flipping or covering to be sure that the top is done.

If you are cooking for several people, be sure to use a large pan. This recipe produces a thick, fluffy omelet. The air you whisked in will insulate the top of the omelet from the cooking heat unless you use a large pan to allow the mixture to spread out.

Energy	127	**calories**
Fat	11	**grams**
Protein	6	**grams**
Carbohydrate	1	**gram**

Main Courses

Fluffy Denver Omelet

1 serving

This uses the recipe for the basic Fluffy Egg Omelet to create a Denver Omelet. The Denver Omelet was first created by Greek immigrant restaurant owners in Denver, giving it a distinct Mediterranean heritage.

Added ingredients	_Amount_
Chopped bell peppers (red, green, or mixed)	1 ounce
Chopped onions	1 ounce
Diced cooked ham or crumbled cooked bacon or sausage	1 ounce
Hot pepper sauce	Optional, to taste

Instructions: Lightly brown the added ingredients in olive oil in the frying pan, then follow the basic Fluffy Egg Omelet recipe *(previous page)* to mix the basic ingredients and slowly stir in the egg mixture. Allow to brown on one side, then, finish by turning it over to brown on the other side. Allow additional time for thicker mixtures when using the fluffy omelet recipe.

The extra ingredients increase the amounts of energy, particularly from protein and carbohydrate in the basic fluffy omelet recipe.

Energy	210	calories
Fat	14	grams
Protein	14	grams
Carbohydrate	7	grams

Pickled Eggs

Serves 12

Prepare in advance and have at hand when needed.

Ingredients	Amount	
Eggs	12	
Vinegar	1	quart
Salt	4	tablespoons
Cayenne pepper	2	tablespoons
Pickling seasoning	2	tablespoons

Instructions: Hard-boil eggs by cooking 20 minutes in simmering water. Cool using cold water, then remove shells. In another pan, add salt and cayenne pepper to vinegar and stir until it comes to a boil. Allow to cool and place into a container with eggs and pickling spice. Cover and set in refrigerator a week before using.

Note: For variety, change spices to allspice and ginger.

If you do home canning, you may want to pour the hot pickling solution over eggs in a heat-resistant glass jar. For your safety, we do not recommend this method, unless you are an experienced canner.

Energy	73	calories
Fat	5	grams
Protein	6	grams
Carbohydrate	1	grams

Quiche

Serves 6

Great choice any time of day.

Ingredients	*Amount*	
Cream	1 ½	cups
Bacon	3	slices
Spinach	10	ounce package, frozen
Shredded cheddar cheese	1	cup
Nutmeg	¼	teaspoon
Basil	1	teaspoon
Eggs	4	
Butter	1	tablespoon

Instructions: Defrost spinach and drain in colander, squeezing as much liquid out as possible. Preheat oven to 325^0. Allow butter to soften to room temperature and use it to coat a 9 inch pie pan. Fry bacon until crisp, remove from frying pan and drain, crumble when cool. Use a saucepan to heat cream, crumbled bacon, and spinach just until boiling. Reduce heat and stir in cheese until cheese is melted. Allow to cool. Add basil and nutmeg. Separate egg whites and beat with an electric mixer until fluffy, then combine with yolks. Slowly stir eggs into cheese mixture. Pour into pie pan and bake 45 minutes. May be served warm or chill in refrigerator and serve cold.

Energy	326	calories
Fat	30	grams
Protein	12	grams
Carbohydrate	2	grams

Fish and Seafood

Eating fish several times a week can be one of the healthiest things you can do. In this section, we have a large number of fish and seafood dishes. However, be aware that not all fish is equally healthy. In general, wild-caught fish are more nutritious than farm-raised fish. Today, much of the fish we eat comes from fish farming. The diet of these pen-raised fish may not be the same as fish in the wild. Fish contain no carbohydrates and always contain protein, but only certain fish contain healthy fish oil. As a general rule, the darker the fish, the more healthy fish oil it contains. Dark varieties of tuna, salmon, herring, and sardines are just some examples.

That does not mean that eating pale colored fish is unhealthy. Light fish, such as whitefish, pollack and tilapia are examples of fish that are practically all protein, but with very little healthy fish oil. If you have one of these as a main course, be sure to balance this high level of protein with additional fat or oil. Similarly, white meat from lobster, shrimp, or crab is essentially pure protein. Balance it with oil or butter.

Beware faux seafood! Imitation crab (sometimes labeled *krab)* and lobster is simply cheap whitefish with artificial flavoring and MSG.

If you wish to use tuna, avoid the inexpensive so-called *tuna in water*. There are many varieties of fish in the tuna family. These generally contain cheaper varieties, are light in color (which means little healthy fish fat) and are packed in a solution labeled as "vegetable broth" (which actually means MSG). Many tuna canners also sell a higher grade fish, packed in olive oil and containing no MSG. Naturally, they charge much more for this variety, but once you taste it, you will never go back.

Baked Catfish in Foil Packets
Serves 4

Moist and tasty!

<u>Ingredient</u>	<u>Amount</u>
Chipotle sauce	1 tablespoon
Ground ginger	1 teaspoon
Olive oil	1 teaspoon
Catfish fillets	4 fillets, about 4 ounces each
Green onion	¼ cup
Sweet red peppers	½ cup
Cucumber	½ cup, peeled and chopped

Instructions: Combine chipotle sauce, ginger and oil, stirring well. Take 4 squares of aluminum foil, about 12 inches each. Place a fish fillet in center of each square. Spoon green onions, pepper and cucumbers evenly over each fillet. Spoon sauce mixture evenly on top. Fold foil over fish to make packets and seal edges tightly. Place packets on baking sheet; bake at 450^0 for 12 minutes. Open packets carefully, as hot steam will escape. Serve.

Energy	130	calories
Fat	4	grams
Protein	19	grams
Carbohydrate	2	grams

Flounder Amandine
Serves 1
A fast gourmet main course.

Ingredients	Amount
Almonds	½ ounce, sliced
Butter	1 teaspoon
Lemon juice	1 teaspoon
Flounder	3 ounces

Instructions: Combine almonds and butter In 9 inch microwavable pie plate. Microwave on high for one minute, stirring once halfway through cooking, until almonds are toasted. Stir in lemon juice. Arrange fish in the bottom of the pie plate and top with almond mixture. Microwave on high for three minutes, let stand one minute before serving.

Energy	192	calories
Fat	12	grams
Protein	19	grams
Carbohydrate	2	grams

Main Courses

Halibut with Mustard Sauce

Serves 1

This tasty dish goes very well with steamed asparagus. The dressing adds flavor and balances the fat-to-protein content.

Ingredients	Amount
Halibut	4 ounce portion
Olive Oil	I to 2 tablespoons
Real Mayonnaise	2 tablespoons
Mustard (powder or prepared)	to taste

Instructions: Cook the halibut in oil in a frying pan or alternatively, broil the fish after brushing with oil. Mix mustard with mayonnaise and top before serving. You may want to vary this recipe by substituting the creamy curry sauce *(page 138)*for the mustard topping.

Energy	345	**calories**
Fat	25	**grams**
Protein	30	**grams**
Carbohydrate	0	**grams**

Latin-Spiced Salmon

Serves 1

Salmon is a food that many recommend eating once or twice a week. This is an easy recipe that brings out its natural flavor. One important ingredient is Tajin®, a powdered Mexican spice often used on fruit. It is MSG-free and contains chili peppers, dehydrated lime and salt. If you cannot find it, experiment with similar ingredients. You should be pleased with the results.

Ingredients	*Amount*
Salmon fillet *(small portion)*	3 ounces *(approximately)*
Olive or sesame oil	1 teaspoon
Tajin™	1 teaspoon, to taste

Instructions: Place fish in baking dish. Brush top of salmon with oil. Sprinkle spice over oil. Place in an oven preheated to 375^{0}F (or 325^{0}F for a convection oven) and cook for 15 to 20 minutes. Check to see that the fish flakes easily with a fork when it appears done.

Alternatively, this may be cooked in a frying pan over medium heat. Use extra oil in the pan and turn once when it is halfway cooked.

Energy	179	calories
Fat	11	grams
Protein	20	grams
Carbohydrate	0	grams

Main Courses

Lemon-Cheese Encrusted Tilapia

Serves 1

Tilapia is a light fish that develops a taste based upon how it is cooked. Since it does not contain much fish oil , frying will help balance the proportion of fat to protein. Its flavor will change, depending upon how it is cooked. Since tilapia fillets are thin, this is an excellent choice for a meal that can be quickly prepared.

Ingredients	Amount	
Tilapia fillets	4	ounces (1 or 2 fillets)
Grated parmesan cheese	1	tablespoon
Dried lemon peel	1	teaspoon
White pepper	½	teaspoon, to taste
Salt		small dash, to taste
Olive or sesame oil		enough to cover pan

Instructions: Grind the dried lemon peel to a powder (using a clean coffee mill or a mortar and pestle) or substitute MSG-free lemon-pepper. Mix the cheese and dry ingredients in a loose bag. Rinse the tilapia fillets and pat on a paper towel so that they are still slightly damp. Coat the fillets completely by shaking them in the bag. Heat the oil to a medium-high temperature before adding the fish. Fry for about 3 to 4 minutes until the crust is brown and crispy on one side. Then turn it over and fry it on the second side until done. Serve immediately.

Energy	232	calories
Fat	15	grams
Protein	23	grams
Carbohydrate	0	grams

Microwave Orange Roughy
Serves 4

A quick dinner meal.

Ingredients	Amount
Orange roughy	1 pound
Cream	¼ cup
Scallions	4
Pepper	To taste
Paprika	To taste

Instructions: Use a microwavable baking dish lightly coated with oil. Place fish in dish and add cream. Chop scallions and sprinkle on top. Microwave for 4 minutes or until fish flakes easily.

Energy	120	calories
Fat	5	grams
Protein	17	grams
Carbohydrate	0	grams

Main Courses

Quick and Creamy Salmon
Serves 2

Fast, easy and delicious.

Ingredients	**Amount**
Salmon	2 filets, 3 to 4 ounces each
Celery	½ cup, chopped
Sour cream	2 tablespoons
Cream	1 tablespoon
Onion	⅛ cup, diced
Garlic salt	To taste
Pepper	To taste
Butter	2 tablespoons

Instructions: Microwave chopped celery and onion in butter for 2 to 3 minutes, in a covered dish on high. Mix in the sour cream, cream, salt, and pepper. Place salmon in the dish, covering with other ingredients. Microwave covered on high for 4 to 5 minutes.

Energy	284	calories
Fat	20	grams
Protein	24	grams
Carbohydrate	2	grams

Seafood Salad
Serves 2

Use a variety of seafood for this delicious cold salad.

Ingredients	Amount	
Cooked seafood	6	ounces
Scallions	¼	cup
Celery	½	cup
Mayonnaise	3	tablespoons
Reduced sugar ketchup	2	teaspoons
Chipotle sauce	1	teaspoon
Wine vinegar	1	teaspoon
Lemon juice	1	teaspoon
White pepper		dash

Instructions: This is a great use for any type of leftover cooked fish. It works well with inexpensive white fish, such as pollack or tilapia, but you can also use real shrimp, lobster or crab. Never use imitation shrimp, lobster, or crabmeat, which are all loaded with MSG. Finely chop the celery and scallions. Mix all the ingredients except the fish well in a large bowl. Cut the cooked fish into cubes, then fold into the mixture. Cover and refrigerate until chilled and you are ready to serve. It can be served on top of a green salad.

Energy	186	**calories**
Fat	18	**grams**
Protein	17	**grams**
Carbohydrate	2	**grams**

Main Courses

Shrimp and Spinach
Serves 4
Bright and colorful main dish.

Ingredients	Amount
Olive oil	2 tablespoons
Minced garlic	1 teaspoon
Shrimp, raw, medium	12 ounces
Crushed red pepper	¼ teaspoon
Spinach, fresh	10 ounces
Grape tomatoes	8
Lemon juice	2 tablespoons

Instructions: Peel and devein the shrimp. Heat oil in a large skillet over medium heat until hot. Add garlic and cook 1 minute, stirring often. Add shrimp and red pepper, cook 2 minutes stirring often. Halve tomatoes. Rinse spinach leaves. Add spinach, tomatoes, lemon juice, ¼ teaspoon salt, and 3 tablespoons water. Cook covered 3 minutes until spinach wilts and shrimp turns pink.

Energy	167	**calories**
Fat	8	**grams**
Protein	19	**grams**
Carbohydrate	4	**grams**

Shrimp in Creamy Mustard Sauce
Serves 3

A quick and delicious meal.

Ingredients	Amount
Cooked and peeled shrimp	1 pound
Onion	¼ cup, chopped *(optional)*
Lemon juice	1 tablespoon
Cream	¼ cup
Prepared mustard	1 tablespoon
Salt and pepper	to taste

Instructions: In a medium-sized saucepan, melt the butter until softened, then add the onion. Stir in lemon juice and bring to a boil. Add cream and lower to a simmer, stirring frequently. Allow to thicken, in about 3 to 4 minutes. Stir in mustard and add shrimp. Continue to cook another 3 to 4 minutes, seasoning with salt and pepper to taste.

Energy	240	calories
Fat	15	grams
Protein	23	grams
Carbohydrate	3	grams

Main Courses

Shrimp in Lemon-Garlic Butter
Serves 4

This Mediterranean-style dish should be served piping hot.

Ingredients	Amount	
Shrimp (uncooked)	1	pound
Olive oil	¼	cup
White pepper	1	teaspoon
Garlic	1	clove
Lemon	1	
Basil	1	tablespoon
Oregano	1	tablespoon
Butter	3	tablespoons

Instructions: Allow butter to soften to room temperature. Put olive oil into a baking dish, use a garlic press to press garlic into dish. Add pepper and mix. Take shrimp and stir or toss in dish so that they are well coated, then distribute evenly. Cut the lemon and squeeze juice over the shrimp, then place the lemon in the dish. Add lemon pieces to the pan. Cover the shrimp with butter, then sprinkle on the basil and oregano. Bake at 375 for 25 minutes, stirring once after 15 minutes. Serve piping hot in baking dish.

Energy	320	calories
Fat	24	grams
Protein	23	grams
Carbohydrate	0	grams

Shrimp Stir-fry

Serves 4

Add an Asian flavor to your meal.

Ingredients	Amount
Precooked shrimp	1 pound
Broccoli, cauliflower, carrot mix	1 12 ounce bag
Olive oil	3 tablespoons
Asian hot oil	½ teaspoon, to taste
Asian five-spice	½ teaspoon, optional

Instructions: Allow frozen vegetables to thaw. Heat oil in a large frying pan or wok. Stir in vegetables and Asian hot oil. Cook about 6 minutes, stirring frequently until softened. Stir in precooked shrimp, heat until warmed.

You may wish to use different mixtures of Asian vegetables and recalculate the nutritional analysis. Remember to never add soy sauce.

Hot oil is an Asian seasoning containing hot pepper extract in a light oil. Five-spice is a ground mixture of anise, cloves, fennel, cinnamon, and pepper. Both can be found in the Asian food section of many supermarkets or at Asian specialty stores.

Energy	227	calories
Fat	12	grams
Protein	24	grams
Carbohydrate	3	grams

Main Courses

Shrimp with Eggplant Kabobs
Serves 2

Intended for use on a barbeque grill, but also can be broiled.

Ingredient	Amount
Butter	1 tablespoon
Large uncooked shrimp	7 ounces
Eggplant	½ cup, cubed
Olive oil	2 teaspoons
Fresh basil	1 tablespoon
Minced garlic	2 cloves
Lemon juice	1 teaspoon

Instructions: Combine all ingredients except shrimp and eggplant in medium bowl and stir. Peel shrimp and cut eggplant into cubes. Add shrimp and eggplant and stir to cover. Cover bowl and refrigerate at least 1 hour or overnight. Preheat grill for 10 minutes. Thread the shrimp and eggplant, alternating, on 2 skewers. Grill or broil, turning occasionally and basting with the remaining marinade. Cook 4 to 6 minutes and serve on skewers

Energy	208	**calories**
Fat	12	**grams**
Protein	21	**grams**
Carbohydrate	4	**grams**

Tilapia with Creamy Shrimp Sauce
Serves 4

This rich dish goes with broccoli or asparagus.

Ingredients	Amount
Precooked small shrimp	4 ounces
Tilapia filets	4 3 ounce filets
Olive oil	1 tablespoon
Salt and black pepper	½ teaspoon each
Whipping cream	¾ cup
Grated parmesan cheese	2 tablespoons
Reduced sugar ketchup	2 tablespoons
White pepper	¼ teaspoon

Instructions: Put cream, ketchup, grated cheese, and white pepper in a medium saucepan and bring to a boil. Next, turn down the heat and simmer for 10 minutes until the sauce starts to thicken. Stir in the shrimp and simmer for 5 more minutes. While this is simmering, place the fish on a foil-lined baking pan, sprinkle with olive oil, then coat with salt and pepper. Broil the fish until it starts to turn brown, which should be approximately five minutes. Put the fish on a serving platter and pour the sauce and shrimp on top.

Energy	257	calories
Fat	16	grams
Protein	25	grams
Carbohydrate	2	grams

Tuna Patties
Serves 2

Serve on a bed of lettuce.

Ingredients	_Amount_
Tuna in olive oil	1 4½ ounce can
Egg	1
Olive oil	1 tablespoon
Celery	¼ cup
Salt and pepper	to taste

Instructions: Chop celery finely. Drain the tuna but save the oil and combine with the olive oil in frying pan. Heat on a medium-high setting. Crumble the tuna. Combine tuna with egg, celery, and spices, mixing well. Fry in oil until brown, turning once.

Energy	154	**calories**
Fat	9	**grams**
Protein	9	**grams**
Carbohydrate	1	**grams**

Grilled Avocado
1 serving

Avocados are high in healthy monounsaturated fat. Most of the carbohydrate they contain is in the form of fiber. Tajin™, a powdered Mexican spice, is MSG-free and contains chili peppers, dehydrated lime, and salt. You may wish to add a small amount of tomato sauce or salsa to the avocado when serving, but remember to add the nutrition information from any added ingredients.

Ingredients	Amount
Avocado	½ per portion
Olive oil	1 teaspoon
Lime or lemon juice	1 teaspoon
Tajin™ or salt and pepper	to taste

Instructions: Slice the avocado in half and remove the seed. Sprinkle oil, juice, and spice in the cavity. Place on hot grill cut side up. Heat a few minutes and serve. You may also want to try cooking this in a frying pan or under a broiler.

Energy	177	calories
Fat	17	grams
Protein	4	grams
Carbohydrate	2	grams

Main Courses

Meat Loaf

Serves 6

This recipe produces a moist, delicious meat loaf. Leftovers can be refrigerated or frozen for later use.

Ingredient	Amount
Ground beef (70/30)	1 pound
Unflavored pork rinds	1 cup (about ¾ oz)
Egg	1
Salt	to taste
Reduced sugar ketchup	2 tablespoons
Mustard	1 teaspoon
Non-calorie brown sugar substitute (Sugar Twin™)	1 tablespoon, to taste

Instructions: Crush the pork rinds into crumbs and mix in a bowl with the meat, egg, and salt. After mixing thoroughly, place in a loaf pan. Combine brown sugar substitute, ketchup and mustard and spread as a topping over the loaf. Bake about 45 to 50 minutes in a 350^0 F. oven (or until internal temperature is at least 150^0 F.). If preparing in a microwave instead, allow about 14 minutes on high before checking temperature.

You may wish to substitute ground pork or MSG-free pork sausage for half the ground beef but recalculate nutrition values. *Cook divided in cupcake tin for easy freezing.*

Energy	230	calories
Fat	16	grams
Protein	18	grams
Carbohydrate	1½	grams

Pasta

Pasta is Italian for paste. It includes all forms of starchy noodles. Obviously, such high carbohydrate products are not appropriate for this plan. Fortunately, there are many creative substitutes that allow familiar dishes to be used.

The lasagna recipe on page 29 is one example. It creates a delicious, layered lasagna without the need for noodles separating the layers. While that approach works for some dishes, others require something with the body of a noodle.

One useful product is spaghetti squash. When fresh spaghetti squash is in season, it can be cooked and the center "spaghetti" strings removed. These are then used just like real spaghetti made from wheat flour.

Another approach is to use *shirataki* (or *shiratake*) noodles, which are made from a Japanese root called *konjac*. These are sometimes referred to as yam noodles, but konjac bears no resemblance to what we would consider a yam.

They produce a noodle that is made of fiber with little protein or carbohydrate content. They have a translucent appearance, looking very similar to Asian rice noodles.

This product is usually sold in a form shaped like cooked spaghetti. However, some of these noodles are now available in other shapes. They require special care in purchasing, handling, cooking and storage. They are always shipped in liquid, sealed in a plastic pouch. They must be kept refrigerated. If purchased from a store, do not buy them if they have been stored without refrigeration. Usually, they are delivered to stores by a refrigerated truck. If purchasing by mail, be certain they did not go without refrigeration for more than one week. Otherwise, they will change consistency and become unusable. Never attempt to freeze them, either before or after cooking. Their consistency will change and they will become tough.

When you'll get ready to use them, open the pouch with scissors. Dump the contents into a colander or strainer in your sink and immediately rinse thoroughly with cold running water. The liquid they were stored in has a fishy odor. Do not worry about it, this will go away with rinsing. Since they are already soft, they need little cooking. Add them to your dish in time for them to warm and flavors to mingle.

This may seem like a lot of trouble, but it will make available to you a whole range of dishes that you thought you could not have while following a plan that was low in carbohydrate. Since these have the consistency of rice noodles, some people find that they are not quite the spaghetti substitute they hoped for. There is a variation of these made with a mixture of konjac and tofu. This has the advantage of being slightly denser and yellow in appearance. This does contain some soy protein. Do not get similar-looking noodles that are made from pure tofu, which are all soy protein.

If your local health food store or Asian market does not carry this product, it is available on the Internet from a wide variety of sources. Some brand names include *Shirakiku*™, *JFC*™, and *Miracle Noodle*™.

When we talk about pasta, people often associate it automatically with tomato sauce. There are many ways to use pasta, without using tomato sauce. Noodles can be blended with olive oil or melted butter, used in a casserole, or served in numerous other ways.

If you wish to be a traditionalist, use your tomato sauce sparingly. Do not forget that tomatoes have a significant amount of carbohydrate, if overused. Never use commercially prepared spaghetti sauce. Instead, make your sauce from fresh or canned tomatoes, adding your own spices and cooking slowly. Commercial sources almost always contain large amounts of MSG and added sugar.

In Italy, there are many white sauces for pasta which contain no tomatoes. When used with shirataki noodles, these are excellent choices for this plan. *Carbonara* sauce is one such example. *Alfredo* sauce is another good choice, but many Alfredo sauce recipes call for a high-carbohydrate thickening agent. The Alfredo sauce recipe on the next page makes a delicious sauce without the carbohydrate thickener.

Alfredo Sauce

Serves 6 (¼ cup servings)

In addition to using this over pasta substitutes, you can also use it as a topping over chicken, shrimp, or vegetables.

Ingredients	**Amount**
Cream	1 cup
Butter	¼ pound (1 stick)
Grated parmesan cheese	¾ cup

Instructions: In a double boiler or on a low heat setting, stir cream and butter till butter is melted and cream is hot. Add parmesan cheese and continue to heat until melted.

For an extra creamy sauce, melt a wedge of original variety Laughing Cow® cheese in the sauce.

Energy	278	**calories**
Fat	28	**grams**
Protein	5	**grams**
Carbohydrate	2	**grams**

Pancakes

Serves 2

Who said you can not have pancakes?

Ingredients	Amount
Almond flour	½ cup
Non-calorie sweetener	6 drops, to taste
Eggs	2
Club soda	⅓ cup
Cream	1 tablespoon
Salt	¼ teaspoon
Cinnamon	dash

Instructions: Beat the eggs and combine all ingredients. Pour into pancakes on a hot, slightly greased griddle or skillet. Turn over once when the bottom is dry. Serve with sugar-free syrup or imitation honey and butter or real whipped cream.

Almond flour is made from ground almonds. It is available in many natural food stores and in some supermarkets.

Energy	240	calories
Fat	21	grams
Protein	12	grams
Carbohydrate	4	gram

Main Courses

Pizza

In recent years, pizza has gone from being a regional ethnic specialty to a national favorite. One legend is that Roman soldiers occupying the Holy Land combined the tomatoes, cheese, and olive oil of their homeland with the flat bread we know today as pita. Whatever its origins, whether you are used to a spongy thick crust or a cracker-like thin crust, people generally love the toppings more than the crust.

Dieters have been creative and submitted many recipes with substitute crusts. We are including one made in a skillet with no crust. The cheese itself holds the ingredients in place. However, you may wish to try other ways.

Some have used the flaxseed bread recipe given on page 126 as a base for their toppings. Others have creatively found ways to bake shirataki noodles into a crust. If affordable, Portabella mushrooms caps also can be used to form a base and hold your other ingredients. Finally, there is the upside-down pizza popularized by a Chicago restaurant. This takes the cheese and sauce and places it in a small crock, just like traditional French onion soup, putting the pizza crust on top. You can use this idea without the top crust!

Remember, tomatoes are high in carbohydrate, so they must be used sparingly.

Pan Pizza

Serves 2

Crustless pizza in a pan.

Ingredients	Amount
Shredded mozzarella	½ cup, real, not from skim milk
Crushed tomatoes	¼ cup
Basil	¼ teaspoon
Oregano	¼ teaspoon
Grated romano cheese	1 tablespoon
Chopped onion	1 tablespoon *(to taste)*
Green pepper	1 tablespoon *(to taste)*
Chopped olives	2 tablespoons *(to taste)*
Sausage *(MSG-free)*	2 ounces

Instructions: Brown crumbled sausage in a small skillet. Drain and set aside. Layer ingredients in the order listed in skillet. Cover with lid and heat on low heat till cheese melts and browns lightly.

Energy	245 calories
Fat	20 grams
Protein	11 grams
Carbohydrate	3 grams

Main Courses

Pork

If you eat pork, you know how it has changed over the years. Traditionally, farm-raised pork was extremely fatty. When the anti-fat hysteria began, pork producers faced a declining market. In response, they totally changed the product. Today, most pork is produced by farmers who contract to large packing companies which provide them pigs to raise. These pigs are selectively bred to be lean and raised with special diets and drugs to provide leaner meat. This creates a high-protein, low-fat product which differs from the balance previously found in pork. The only way that I know to get old-fashioned pork products is to buy them directly from a small farmer selling heritage-variety pork at a farmers' market.

This is not a problem if you are using some of the fattier cuts. These will work fine if you cook them in your traditional way. However, if you are using lean chops with little visible fat, balance the fat content of your meals through another dish or a topping. As an example, brush lean pork chops with olive oil and sprinkle them with Tajin® before baking, broiling or pan-frying in the usual manner. Another topping to use before baking is a mixture of mayonnaise and mustard, which gives a luscious and juicy result.

If you buy large roasts, try to avoid those in sealed packages with liquid and chemicals added. Whatever you do, avoid commercially prepared barbecue sauce. Instead, try our barbecue and meat sauce recipe on page 135.

Picante Pork Chops

Serves 1

A slow-cooked recipe that works for some of the tougher cuts. Multiply this recipe by the number of portions desired.

Ingredients	Amount
Pork chop	4 ounces
Picante sauce	4 tablespoons *(MSG and sugar-free)*

Instructions: Brown chop in skillet on both sides. Pour some sauce into an electric Crock-Pot®, add chop and top with remaining sauce. Cover and cook on low heat for 10 hours or on the high setting for 3 to 4 hours.

Energy	185	calories
Fat	9	grams
Protein	22	grams
Carbohydrate	4	grams

Main Courses

Poultry

Poultry used to be a special treat, but today, mass-production farms have turned chicken into an everyday dish. Unfortunately, the anti-fat hysteria has caused producers to give us poultry products such as turkeys bred to have lots of breast meat and little leg meat. Heritage breeds still exist, usually from small farmers raising them for gourmet and specialty shops. Most of the time, you will have to make do with what is available you locally.

Since you are not avoiding using poultry to avoid fat, here are some suggestions. Consider using dark meat instead of white meat whenever possible. Thighs and drumsticks work well. Leave the skin on. The layer of fat found under the skin will add flavor to the poultry and will help balance the protein found in the muscle. Try to avoid injected meat, such as the self-basting turkeys advertised around holiday time. If possible, do not buy products with retained fluid. Supermarket chicken today is loaded with a mixture of water and chemicals. You can avoid this if you can get chicken that is truly fresh directly from a farmer. One national brand, *Smart Chicken*®, contains no added water or chemicals. It is available in many supermarkets. (C*heck www.SmartChicken.com to locate a retailer near you.*)

You may use most of your traditional methods of cooking poultry. Substitute grated cheese or crushed pork rinds for breading. Use any of the chicken recipes that follow to add variety to your meals.

Baked Chicken

Serves 6

You may find this easy and delicious dish is better than fried.

Ingredients	Amount
Chicken legs	2 pounds
Grated parmesan cheese	½ cup
Poultry seasoning	1 teaspoon *(msg-free)*
Paprika	2 ½ teaspoons
Garlic powder	½ teaspoon
Pepper	¼ teaspoon

Instructions: Wash chicken but leave moist. Place other ingredients in a plastic bag and mix together. Add chicken and shake the bag well to coat the chicken pieces. Place the chicken in a shallow pan and bake at 350 for 60 minutes.

You may vary or substitute the spices to your taste. Consider using crushed pork rinds as an additional coating.

Energy	241	calories
Fat	16	grams
Protein	23	grams
Carbohydrate	1	grams

Main Courses

Chicken *Mole*

1 serving

Mole, pronounced ***mo-lay***, is a Mexican dish, which has many regional variations. It contains chocolate, ground nuts, chili pepper, other spices and sweetener. This recipe does not claim authenticity but it is tasty. Vary it as you like. It works well with other dishes besides chicken, too.

Ingredients	**Amount**
Chicken breast	½ portion, about 4 ounces
Olive oil	2 tablespoons
100% cocoa powder	1 teaspoon
Cinnamon	½ teaspoon, to taste
Liquid non-calorie sweetener	1 teaspoon, to taste
Hot pepper sauce	½ teaspoon, to taste
Natural peanut butter	1 teaspoon, to taste
Ground red pepper	½ teaspoon, to taste

Instructions: Cook chicken by sautéing it in oil in a frying pan. Lower heat to simmer and mix in other ingredients. Stir to mix as peanut butter softens. Add a little water or MSG-free chicken broth to thin, if needed. Cover and simmer for a few minutes to allow flavors to mix. Add other ingredients, such as sliced mushrooms, if desired. You may also want to try this as a meat or chicken stir-fry, featuring cut-up leftovers and vegetables.

Energy	178	calories
Fat	18	grams
Protein	27	grams
Carbohydrate	2	grams

Chicken Salad

Serves 4

Nice luncheon dish.

Ingredients	*Amount*
Mayonnaise	½ cup
Sour cream	½ cup
Unsweetened dill relish	1 tablespoon
Diced chicken	1 cup
Diced celery	½ cup
Salt	to taste
Pepper	to taste

Instructions: Mix mayonnaise, sour cream, and relish together in a small bowl. Mix diced chicken and diced celery together in large bowl. Add the mayonnaise mixture to the chicken mixture, adding salt and pepper to taste. Cover and chill for at least 2 hours to let flavors blend.

Energy	388	**calories**
Fat	38	**grams**
Protein	12	**grams**
Carbohydrate	3	**grams**

Chicken with Creamy Mustard Sauce
Serves 4

A tasty pan-fried dish.

Ingredients	*Amount*	
Prepared mustard	2	teaspoons
Mayonnaise	2	teaspoons
Lime juice	1	teaspoons
Olive oil	1	teaspoon
Chicken legs	4	

Instructions: Combine mustard, mayonnaise, and lime juice, and stir well. Heat oil in a frying pan and add chicken. Cover and cook 12 to 15 minutes until chicken is cooked, using medium heat and turning once. Remove chicken and place on serving platter. Add mustard mixture to pan drippings and stir. Spoon mixture over chicken and serve.

Energy	375	calories
Fat	27	grams
Protein	31	grams
Carbohydrate	0	grams

Hearty Chicken Stew

Serves 4

This is too thick and rich to call chicken soup. Stew is a much better description for this hearty main course. It bears no resemblance to those MSG-laden canned broths, but might resemble something recognizable by your great-grandparents.

Ingredient	_Amount_	
Chicken leg quarter	1	about 1 lb
Water	10	cups
Celery	2	stalks
Carrots	2	
Old Bay™ seasoning (or celery salt or celery seed)		to taste (MSG-free original formula)
Salt and pepper		to taste
Onion		to taste
Mushroom pieces	1	4 ounces can

Instructions: Use a large pot or an electric Crock-Pot® or slow cooker. Remove any attached organs from the chicken but leave the skin and fat on. Cut the celery and carrots into pieces about ½ inch long. Place all ingredients but the mushrooms into the pot and bring it to a boil.

Reduce heat to a simmer and cover loosely. Allow to simmer several hours. If you are using a Crock-Pot®, it is fine to leave it on all day or overnight on a low setting. Cook until the meat is literally falling off the bones.

Allow it to cool enough to safely handle. Use a strainer, colander, or ladle to separate the solids from the broth and then carefully pick out and discard all the bones.

continued on next page

Hearty Chicken Stew - continued

Take out all the skin and fat and about half of the meat, place it in an electric blender or food processor and purée to a thick consistency. Return all ingredients to the pot, add the mushrooms, bring it back to a boil, and let it cook, uncovered until you are ready to serve. For a thick and hearty stew, this should reduce the volume to about 4 cups.

If you want to serve this as a lighter soup, begin with more water or do not reduce it quite as much. You may also want to save some of the clear broth as a base for other soup recipes.

Energy	257	calories
Fat	17	grams
Protein	20	grams
Carbohydrate	5	grams

Chicken with Lemon

Serves 6

This roast chicken makes a nice Sunday dinner.

Ingredients	Amount
Chicken	3 pounds
Tarragon	2 teaspoons
Salt	½ teaspoon
Lemon	1
Pepper	½ teaspoon

Instructions: Preheat oven to 350^0, rinse chicken with cold water, and dry with paper towel. Combine tarragon, salt, and pepper and rub mixture over chicken. Place cut up lemon in chicken cavity, secured with toothpicks. Coat baking dish or pan with oil or spray, and bake at 350^0 approximately 1½ hours or until the internal temperature is 180^0 F. Cover with foil and let stand about 15 minutes. Remove and discard lemon.

Energy	338	calories
Fat	23	grams
Protein	29	grams
Carbohydrate	2	grams

Spicy Chicken Wings
Serves 4

A great meal or snack while watching football.

Ingredients	_Amount_	
Chicken wings	1½	pounds
Chipotle sauce	⅓	cup
Liquid sweetener	½	teaspoon
Water	½	cup
Garlic powder	½	teaspoon
Pepper		to taste

Instructions: Rinse chicken. Cut up pieces, if desired. Place in large bowl. Combine remaining ingredients and pour over chicken. Marinate in refrigerator for 4 hours. Place chicken and sauce in baking dish coated with nonstick spray. Bake 35 to 40 minutes until chicken is thoroughly cooked.

Consider serving these with bleu cheese dressing and celery sticks.

Energy	209	calories
Fat	15	grams
Protein	17	grams
Carbohydrate	1	grams

Spicy Lime Chicken
Serves 4

Tajin® is a wonderful Mexican spice combining lime, red pepper, and salt.

Ingredients	Amount
Skinless chicken breast	2 pounds
Olive oil	1 tablespoon
Lime juice	1 teaspoon
Tajin®	2 teaspoons

Instructions: Cut chicken into 4 portions. Mix olive oil and lime juice. Brush both sides of the chicken with mixture and place it in baking dish or pan. Sprinkle Tajin® over the chicken. Bake at 350^0 for about 40 minutes and serve.

.

Energy	130	calories
Fat	5	grams
Protein	21	grams
Carbohydrate	0	grams

Main Courses

Salads

Salads are not new to dieting. One question is whether to consider salads a main course, a side dish, an accompaniment, or a snack? The answer is yes to each of these, since a salad can be anything you want it to be, depending upon size and content.

There is one important caveat. It was well understood for almost a century that the dressing was more important than the salad itself. In the last few decades, as part of the anti-fat hysteria, this has been forgotten. People developed a magical belief that it was the salad itself and healthy dressings were a no-no. Think of a salad as a good place to hold salad dressing. The commercially available bottled "salad dressings", particularly those labeled "low fat," are of no help to the dieter. Often, they are loaded with sugar and MSG and have the opposite effect you desire.

Get back to basics! Olive oil, the traditional dressing for your salad greens, is still the best choice. If you find extra-virgin olive oil too heavy for your taste, try using unrefined sesame oil, the choice suggested by Hippocrates 2,400 years ago. You may add salt and pepper to taste. Add vinegar if you choose; it is optional. Use any form of vinegar except balsamic vinegar. Balsamic vinegar starts out as ordinary wine vinegar, which is then modified with the addition of grape sugars after the vinegar has been produced.

Another forgotten dressing for salad is real mayonnaise. If this seems too bland for you, dress it up with other ingredients. One old-style recipe is adding a dash of ketchup to mayonnaise for a so-called Russian dressing. Just remember to use low-carbohydrate ketchup.

Salad greens themselves are leafy plants. Use any of the various types of lettuce that you prefer. Generally, they all work well. Lettuces contain a small amount of carbohydrate, some fiber, and some water. If you were to eat nothing but lettuce, you could gain weight, based on the carbohydrates. However, balancing the lettuce with the healthy fat of olive oil or sesame oil is the real benefit. The carbohydrate content is normally low enough to be a small part of your allowance. This is the type of food you should be saving your carbohydrate allowance for every day. Cabbage is little denser in carbohydrate and can be used, but more sparingly.

You might try adding a flowery vegetable, such as raw broccoli or cauliflower as a garnish. Avoid any higher carbohydrate items, such as beans and peas. Tomatoes are high in carbohydrates, so use them very small amounts, such as one or two grape tomatoes.

If you would like to make this salad more of a meal, consider adding a bit of leftover meat or chicken or a few strips of canned fish such as sardines or kippered herrings. Slices of hard-boiled egg or crumbled cheese also work. If this is beginning to sound like a chef's salad or a Cobb salad, you're correct. Adding this protein in small amounts to the salad works very well to produce a complete meal. Additional flavor may also be added with avocado, which is primarily fat. You can vary the type of salad you have and have a wide range of choices.

Size matters. Keep the size of your salad down to a small dinner salad, such as you might put in a small soup bowl. You may want to start out using pre-washed bagged lettuce, simply because the nutritional analysis is on the package. Until you become accustomed to the right size salad, this is an easy method of letting you estimate the content of your salads. If you have a chef's salad at a typical restaurant, it will be about three times the size you would make at home. Share it with friends.

The recipe that follows is for a tasty dinner salad. Chapter 7 has some additional dressing recipes you may enjoy.

Egg, Bacon, and Avocado Salad
Serves 6

A filling meal for all.

Ingredient	_Amount_	
Romaine lettuce	1	head
Bacon	8	slices
Avocados	2	
Eggs	4	
Tomato	1	medium size
Crumbled bleu cheese	4	ounces
Dressing ingredients		
Garlic clove	1	crushed *(optional)*
Liquid sweetener	6	drops, to taste
Lemon Juice	2	tablespoons
Olive oil	¼	cup
Salt and pepper		to taste

Instructions: Fry bacon until crisp, then crumble. Hard-boil eggs, cool, shell and chop. Wash and slice or tear lettuce, and then arrange on a large platter. Peel and dice the avocado. Chop the tomato. Place all these over the lettuce, with bacon on top. Combine dressing ingredients in a jar and shake well. Pour over salad and serve.

Energy	330	calories
Fat	28	grams
Protein	13	grams
Carbohydrate	6	grams

Stuffed Peppers

Many ethnic traditions include dishes with meat baked in pepper shells. Some classic recipes use a carbohydrate filler, such as rice. By eliminating the carbohydrate filler, these tasty dishes may be adapted to this diet. A few recipes follow, but you can be inventive and create your own. One example might be to use the meat loaf recipe baked in a green pepper shell.

Cream Cheese and Bacon-Stuffed Jalapeno
Serves 1

This dish works as either a main course or a party snack

Ingredients	Amount
Jalapeno Peppers	3
Cream cheese	2 ounces
Bacon	2 slices
Salt and pepper	To taste

Instructions: Cut the tops off of the peppers. Slice the peppers in half, lengthwise, and clean out the seeds and membranes. Divide cream cheese into six parts and spread one part into each hollowed-out pepper. Press one third of a slice of bacon into the cream cheese in each pepper. Season with salt and pepper to taste. Place on a greased cookie sheet. Bake about 25 minutes at 350^0 until bacon is cooked through.

For crisper bacon, partially cook the bacon first.

Energy	184	calories
Fat	26	grams
Protein	9	grams
Carbohydrate	3	grams

Sausage Stuffed Jalapeños
Serves 4

Another main course that also works as a party snack.

Ingredients	Amount	
Pork sausage (*MSG-free*)	1	pound
Cream cheese	8	ounces
Shredded parmesan cheese	1	cup
Jalapeño peppers	20	
Ground cumin		to taste
Ground red pepper		to taste

Instructions: Halve the peppers lengthwise and clean out. Crumble the sausage and brown in a large skillet with the ground red pepper and cumin. Drain excess grease, then combine with the cheeses. Divide mixture, spooning about 1 tablespoon into each pepper half. Place into lightly greased baking pans. Bake at 425 degrees for 15 to 20 minutes, until lightly browned.

Energy	283	calories
Fat	26	grams
Protein	9	grams
Carbohydrate	2	grams

Stuffed Green Peppers
Serves 4

A traditional dish, with a change of filler.

Ingredient	Amount
Green bell peppers	2
Ground beef	8 ounces
Grated Swiss cheese	2 ounces
Pork rinds, unflavored	½ ounce
Salt and pepper	To taste

Instructions: Place pork rinds in a plastic bag and crush to a powder. Mix with beef, salt, and pepper. Halve peppers lengthwise and clean out. Divide meat mixture and place in hollowed-out peppers. Top with cheese. Place about a quarter inch of water into a baking dish. Carefully arrange the peppers side-by-side and bake about 45 minutes in a 375° oven, until peppers are soft and meat is thoroughly cooked.

Energy	265	calories
Fat	20	grams
Protein	16	grams
Carbohydrate	3	grams

Wraps

Wraps are another special main course option. There are no specific recipes here for wraps. Instead, they are simply suggested, allowing you to use your imagination and creativity for the filling.

Many restaurants now offer wraps as a standard item or an alternative to sandwiches. They often contain a mixture of salad and meat or breakfast items.

The diet issue is the wrapper. When you make your wraps, select a low-carbohydrate item for the wrapper. Raw lettuce leaves or lightly steamed cabbage leaves may work well. Low-carbohydrate tortilla shells can also be used.

If you prefer your tortilla wrapper crunchier, fry it. After filling your wrap, briefly fry it in a frying pan with a small amount of oil. This will make the wrapper crispy, like a taco shell.

Chapter 3

Side Dishes

Side dishes accompany the main course of a meal. Are they necessary? At times, they are vital to give balance to a meal. At other times, such as when serving a casserole as a main dish, they may be unnecessary. Part of meal planning is deciding what side dish should accompany a particular main course, both to balance the meal nutritionally and to meet your tastes.

Alternatively, sometimes a side dish may be all that you want. That is perfectly all right, as long as you are getting the proper balance. At times, just having a simple dinner salad to accompany the main course will be perfect.

Whether your side dish is simply a salad or a cooked vegetable, it is usually a vegetable dish of some sort. You do not need a recipe for simply cooking a vegetable or serving a dinner salad. The important thing here is making the right choice. Fresh, in-season vegetables are always an excellent choice, but remember to stick to the low-carbohydrate leaves and flowers of the plant. Think about using broccoli asparagus, and cauliflower. Avoid all the high-carbohydrate root vegetables such as potatoes and beets. If you are using frozen vegetables, avoid the ones that come seasoned or with their own sauce.

Depending on the vegetable you choose, there are a variety of cooking methods available. You do not need to be limited to just boiling or microwaving your vegetables. Think about lightly steaming, baking, broiling, frying, or even grilling. In some situations, you might think about adding flavor by brushing your vegetables with olive oil and then sprinkling on coarse salt or spices.

In addition to the simple vegetable side dishes just discussed, the recipes that follow provide some ideas that may be for special occasions or for everyday use.

Cauliflower "Mashed Potatoes"
Serves 4

If you like mashed potatoes, you will love this rich and creamy side dish. *You may want to experiment, reducing ingredients to achieve ideal consistency. This is very tasty, so do not overdo your portion size.*

<u>Ingredients</u>	<u>Amount</u>
Fresh or frozen cauliflower	8 ounces (½ bag)
Cream	¼ cup
Butter	3 tablespoons
Cream cheese	4 ounces (½ package)

Instructions: Cook cauliflower by steaming, boiling, or microwaving until well done and soft. Drain well in a colander and squeeze out remaining water until very dry. Soften butter to room temperature or in microwave. Put into food processor and run, adding other ingredients as you go, adding cream last to control the consistency. Run until creamy and smooth. Serve warm, reheating if needed.

Optional: Top with grated cheese, but add to the totals

Energy	226 calories
Fat	22 grams
Protein	4 grams
Carbohydrate	3 grams

Side Dishes

Cauliflower "Potato Salad"

4 servings

Your guests may prefer this to traditional potato salad.

Ingredients	*Amount*
Cauliflower	1 frozen bag (5 cups)
Celery stalks	2
Hard-boiled eggs	2
Celery seed	½ teaspoon
Mayonnaise	¼ cup
Cream	2 tablespoon
Lemon juice	2 tablespoon
Dry mustard	½ teaspoon
Liquid non-calorie sweetener	1 tablespoon or to taste
Prepared mustard	1 tablespoon
Salt and pepper	to taste
Nutmeg	optional, to taste

Instructions: Steam cauliflower about 10 minutes or until tender. Allow to cool, then cut into bite-size pieces. Chop celery into bite size pieces. Remove shells from hard-boiled eggs after allowing them to cool. Slice in egg slicer, after cutting the egg in half lengthwise or chop into small pieces. Combine all ingredients, cover, and refrigerate until chilled.

Energy	209	calories
Fat	17	**grams**
Protein	7	**grams**
Carbohydrate	6	**grams**

Chilled Marinated Asparagus
4 servings

A good side dish with salmon.

<u>Ingredients</u>	<u>Amount</u>
Asparagus	1 pound
Liquid non-calorie sweetener	2 teaspoons
Cider vinegar	⅓ cup
Olive oil	⅓ cup
Lemon juice	2 teaspoons

Instructions: Combine all ingredients except asparagus and mix well. In a large skillet, bring ½ inch of water to a boil. Add asparagus and reduce heat to a simmer. Cover and cook 3 to 5 minutes. Drain and rinse in cold water. Place asparagus in a large resealable plastic bag and add marinade. Seal the bag and turn to coat. Refrigerate for several hours, turning occasionally. Drain and discard the excess marinade. Place asparagus on a serving plate.

Consider topping with the Creamy Curry Sauce found on page138.

Energy	178 calories
Fat	9 grams
Protein	1 grams
Carbohydrate	3 grams

Cole Slaw

Serves 4

A traditional summertime and picnic favorite.

Ingredients	*Amount*
Shredded cabbage	2 cups
Mayonnaise	6 tablespoons
Cream	4 tablespoons
Liquid sweetener	½ teaspoon, to taste
Salt	¼ teaspoon, to taste
Pepper	¼ teaspoon, to taste
Lemon juice	2 teaspoon, to taste

Instructions: Combine all ingredients except cabbage in a large bowl. Beat with electric beater or whisk until creamy. Fold in shredded cabbage and mix well with a large spoon. Cover and refrigerate until chilled.

Energy	**193 calories**
Fat	**21 grams**
Protein	**1 grams**
Carbohydrate	**1 grams**

Country Fried Cabbage

Serves 4

Great side dish.

Ingredients	*Amount*
Shredded cabbage	3 cups
Butter	2 tablespoons
Vinegar	1 tablespoon
Cream	2 tablespoons
Water	2 tablespoons, as needed
Salt and pepper	To taste

Instructions: Melt the butter in a large skillet then add cabbage. Stir over medium heat until slightly browned. Lower heat, cover and cook until cabbage is tender. Stir in vinegar and cream, with water, as needed, and heat thoroughly. Season with salt and pepper

Energy	83	calories
Fat	8	grams
Protein	1	grams
Carbohydrate	2	grams

Creamed Mushrooms

Serves 4

Goes great with steak.

Ingredients	Amount
Butter	2 tablespoons
Mushrooms (sliced)	1 ½ cups
Paprika	½ teaspoon
Sour cream	8 tablespoons

Instructions: Melt butter. Add mushrooms and sauté over low heat for approximately 10 minutes. Add paprika and stir. Cover, turn off heat and allow to cool 5 minutes. Add sour cream a little at a time and stir after each addition

Energy	57	**calories**
Fat	5	**grams**
Protein	1	**gram**
Carbohydrate	2	**grams**

Creamed Spinach

Serve 4

Serve with chicken or salmon for a complete meal.
Substitute different cheeses for variety.

Ingredient	Amount
Spinach, frozen	1 bag, 12 ounces
Butter	2 tablespoons
Cream	½ cup
Shredded Swiss cheese	¾ cup
Salt and pepper	To taste

Instructions: Allow spinach to thaw or microwave about 3 minutes. Melt butter in large pan, then add thawed spinach. Cook on low heat, stirring occasionally, until most liquid has evaporated. Add cream and cheese. Use salt and pepper to taste. Stir until the cheese has melted and serve hot.

Energy	268	calories
Fat	22	grams
Protein	7	grams
Carbohydrate	3	grams

Italian Broccoli and Tomatoes
Serves 4

Goes well with salmon or pork.

<u>Ingredients</u>	<u>Amount</u>
Broccoli	½ pound
Grape tomatoes	8
Water	1 tablespoon
Garlic powder	¼ teaspoon *(optional)*
Oregano	¼ teaspoon
Shredded mozzarella cheese	¼ cup
Sliced black olives	1 tablespoon

Instructions: Lightly steam or boil broccoli 5 to 8 minutes until just tender. Drain and place broccoli in a saucepan. Halve the grape tomatoes. Add tomatoes, water, garlic powder, and oregano and stir gently. Cook uncovered, over medium-low heat until thoroughly heated, stirring occasionally. Sprinkle with cheese and olives. Remove from heat. Cover and let stand 2 to 3 minutes, until cheese melts.

Energy	**42 calories**
Fat	**2 grams**
Protein	**4 grams**
Carbohydrate	**2 grams**

Slow-Cooked Mushrooms

Serves 16

Use this as a party appetizer or freeze in individual portions as a side-dish.

Ingredients	Amount
Fresh small mushrooms	4 pounds
Butter	½ pound
Chipotle sauce	1 tablespoon
Dill seed	½ teaspoon
Pepper	½ teaspoon
Garlic powder	½ teaspoon
Home-made chicken stock	1 quart

Instructions: Wash the mushrooms, and trim the stem ends. Combine with all other ingredients in a large covered stock pot or a Crock-Pot®. Cover and simmer on low or medium-low heat for 5 to 6 hours or overnight. Gently stir occasionally. Remove lid and cook uncovered for another 3 to 6 hours or until liquid has reduced to barely cover mushrooms. Serve in a chafing dish with toothpicks as an appetizer, or use as a side dish. These freeze well and may be reheated in a saucepan over low heat or in the microwave.

Energy	128 calories
Fat	12 grams
Protein	2 grams
Carbohydrate	3 grams

Side Dishes

Sour Cream Cucumbers
Serves 8

Refreshing summertime side-dish.
Keeps well in refrigerator.

Ingredients	Amount
Large cucumbers	2
Large onion	1
Sour cream	¾ cup
Cider vinegar	3 tablespoons
Liquid non-calorie sweetener	1 teaspoon
Salt and pepper	To taste

Instructions: Peel and slice the cucumbers. Peel the onion and slice into rings. Place the cucumbers and onions in a large container. Combine the remaining ingredients and pour over cucumbers. Mix well and cover. Chill in the refrigerator.

Energy	62	calories
Fat	5	grams
Protein	1	grams
Carbohydrate	4	grams

Spiced Zucchini
Serves 4

Serve with fish or chicken.

Ingredients	Amount
Olive oil	1 tablespoon
Whole cumin seed	1 teaspoon
Zucchini	1 ½ pounds
Salt and pepper	To taste

Instructions: Heat oil over medium-high heat in a large skillet. Add cumin seeds. Cook about 30 seconds, stirring constantly until fragrant and sizzling. Add zucchini, which has been cut into ½ inch slices. Reduce heat to medium and cook 6 to 7 minutes, stirring occasionally until lightly browned and tender. Season with salt and pepper. Serve.

Energy	54	calories
Fat	4	grams
Protein	2	grams
Carbohydrate	3	grams

Squash Sauté

Serves 4

An inexpensive dish when squash is in season.

Ingredients	Amount
Green and yellow squash	4 cups
Garlic	2 cloves *(optional)*
Olive oil	1 tablespoon
Shredded mozzarella cheese	½ cup
Fresh basil	2 tablespoons
Salt and pepper	To taste

Instructions: Slice squash. Peel and mince garlic. Add basil. Sauté together in olive oil, in a frying pan, until the squash is soft. Add cheese, stir and allow the cheese to melt. Serve.

Energy	99	**calories**
Fat	7	**grams**
Protein	5	**grams**
Carbohydrate	4	**grams**

Zucchini Hash Browns
Serves 4

Not quite the same as potatoes.

Ingredient	Amount
Grated zucchini	1 cup
Grated onion	2 tablespoons
Eggs	2
Salt and pepper	To taste
Garlic powder	To taste
Olive oil	2 tablespoons

Instructions: Heat oil in a heavy skillet. Lightly beat eggs and mix with remaining ingredients. Drop heaping tablespoons in hot oil, turning when brown. Keep cooked zucchini on a plate in a warm oven until entire batch is done, then serve.

If you wish, top with sour cream or butter, but add these to the nutritional totals.

Energy	103	calories
Fat	9	grams
Protein	4	grams
Carbohydrate	2	grams

Chapter 4

Soups

Soups can accompany a meal or they can be the meal itself. Whether it is a warm bowl of soup on a cold winter evening or a chilled soup on a summer afternoon, a cozy bowl of soup can bring back fond memories. Some soups are so rich that they defy the definition of an accompaniment. That's why the hearty chicken stew recipe on page 73 is listed as a main course, instead of putting it in this chapter.

Avoid commercial soups! Canned soup manufacturers have long since turned to MSG to improve the taste of their soup. Today, at least in the United States, some soup producers even attempt to advertise that they are free of MSG when, in fact, they are loaded with it. Powdered and packaged soups are even worse. Have you ever wondered how they can get all that chicken flavor in a small bouillon cube? For the few pennies that it costs, do you think a chicken ever got near the soup factory?

At one time, everyone made his or her own soups. That required longer hours at the stove and careful watching. Perhaps it was the long hours of attention that made soup-making less practical in today's modern home. The good news is that electric Crock-Pots® and slow cookers have make homemade soup practical again. They require little attention while they simmer for hours, bringing out the full flavor of the soups' natural ingredients.

Many soup recipes use cheap carbohydrate fillers. Obviously, that is not appropriate on this diet. Think about it for moment, and you will realize that the carbohydrate fillers were substitutes for the natural ingredients. As an example, when was the last time you had a seafood chowder that was made with real cream instead of potatoes? When was the last time you had chicken soup made from real chicken rather than starting with a semi-artificial chicken stock? Again, it's a question of getting back to basics.

Some soups are harder to make today, because real ingredients are hard to find. When people bought their meat directly from a butcher, the bones were sold or given free to the customer for making soup. These soups bones produced a rich flavor and the marrow was a source of many nutrients. Today when butchering is done at distant plants, most of the bones are ground up for animal feed.

Once you relearn the lost art of making soup, I doubt that you will ever want to go back to eating the other product. Hopefully the few recipes we have included here will be a good start.

Asparagus Soup

Serves 7

A tasty treat when asparagus are in season.
The unused portions freeze well

Ingredient	*Amount*
Chicken stock, *MSG-free*	2½ cups
Asparagus	1¼ pounds
Cream	½ cup
Water	1½ cups
Salt and pepper	to taste

Instructions: Cut asparagus into inch-long pieces. Combine ingredients and cook slowly for several hours to allow the flavors to blend.

Be sure to use a homemade chicken stock or one you are certain *is free of MSG. Some brands that advertise that they are MSG-free contain fine print, which states that they actually do contain MSG.* **Read the fine print.**

Energy	76 calories
Fat	6 grams
Protein	2 grams
Carbohydrate	2 grams

Soups

Chicken Noodle Soup
Serves 6

Hearty enough to be a main course. Well worth the effort.

Ingredients	Amount	
Chicken leg quarters	2	
Water	6	cups
Carrots	1½	medium
Celery (diced)	1 ½	cups
Salt	1	teaspoon
Pepper	¼	teaspoon
Shirataki* yam noodles	1	package

Instructions: Put chicken in large stockpot. Cover with water and bring to a boil. Skim top. Reduce to simmer, and cook with a tight lid for 2 hours. Peel and slice carrots and add, along with celery, salt, and pepper. Return to a boil, then cover and lower heat. Simmer for 1 hour. Remove chicken and debone it. Remove the skin. Chop the chicken and return 3 cups of chopped chicken to the pot, saving the rest for another use. Simmer on low. Cut open the package of shirataki over a colander or strainer, in the sink, drain off liquid and rinse thoroughly for about two minutes. Add noodles to soup and cook for an additional 30 minutes. Add additional salt to taste. *You may store this soup in the refrigerator but do not freeze it.*

*__*Note:__ Shirataki noodles are discussed in detail on page 59. They have virtually no calories and work well in soups.*

Energy	79	**calories**
Fat	5	**grams**
Protein	6	**grams**
Carbohydrate	2	**grams**

Cream of Cauliflower Soup
Serves 4

A rich taste you never could find in a can.

<u>Ingredients</u>	<u>Amount</u>
Celery	2 stalks
Cauliflower	1 cup
Garlic	1 clove *(optional)*
Water	1 cup
Salt and pepper	to taste
Cayenne pepper	dash
Chicken stock, *MSG-free*	⅔ cup
Cream	⅓ cup

Instructions: Dice celery and mince garlic. Combine with cauliflower, water, salt, and cayenne pepper in a medium pot. Bring to a boil, then lower to a simmer for 15 minutes. Carefully transfer to a blender. Cover and blend at high speed, until pureed. Return to the pot, adding the broth and cream. Reheat for 10 to 15 minutes and serve hot. Season with black pepper to taste.

*Be sure to use a homemade chicken stock or one you are <u>certain</u> is free of MSG. Some brands that advertise that they are MSG-free contain fine print, which states that they actually do contain MSG. **Read the fine print.***

Energy	85	calories
Fat	8	grams
Protein	2	grams
Carbohydrate	2	grams

Roasted Red Pepper Soup

Serves 4

You will need a food processor to make this delicious soup.

Ingredient	_Amount_
Red peppers	3 medium size
Cream	½ cup
Sour cream	8 tablespoons
Olive oil	1 tablespoon
Thyme	1 tablespoon
Water	1 cup
Garlic	2 cloves (optional)
Salt and pepper	To taste

Instructions: Cut peppers lengthwise, then remove and discard the seeds and inside membrane. Flatten peppers and place skin side up in a baking pan. Place under broiler, about 2 to 3 inches from the heat and cook until the skin is blackened. Remove peppers and place in a bowl of cold water to cool. Once cool, peel and discard the skins. Mince the garlic. Place all ingredients, except the sour cream, into a food processor and process until smooth. Pour the mixture into a saucepan and adjust the heat as necessary, cooking until the soup thickens and is bubbly. Top each portion with 2 tablespoons of sour cream when serving.

Energy	188	calories
Fat	17	grams
Protein	2	grams
Carbohydrate	6	grams

Chapter 5

Beverages

What you drink can be an important factor in weight-control. Today, carbonated, sugar-laden and caffeinated beverages are an unfortunate part of the typical diet for many Americans. People need fluid in their diet and the obvious answer is pure water. Ultimately, in any diet, that should be your goal. However, custom, habit and taste may play a large part in influencing you.

Although had the soft-drink craze is fairly recent in human history, an aversion to water is not. There are records of beer production in ancient Mesopotamia. Both the Bible and historical records, tell us about ancient use of wine. One important note is that those alcoholic beverages, often diluted with water, helped sanitize contaminated water supplies and may have prevented outbreaks of disease. The more that people began to live closely together in cities and villages, the more likely they were to use contaminated water supplies. It is only in the 20th century that Americans and most Europeans could drink tap water that was free from bacterial contamination.

Today, in the United States, tap water

contaminated by bacteria is virtually unknown. However, in some locales, chemical contamination is become a concern, either because of health risks or peculiar odors and taste.

If you live in an area where the local tap water is unpleasant, add a filter to your tap or use a filter pitcher. These are inexpensive ways to remove contaminants and improve your water's taste.

There has been a tremendous upsurge in the sales of bottled water, for the same reason. There is criticism of bottled water, due to the environmental impact of disposable bottles and transportation of water. However if bottled water is replacing bottled soda, its environmental impact is no worse than the product it replaced.

If you have become accustomed to beverages other than water, you may not want to make this switch to water or do it gradually over time. Therefore, it is practical to think about the beverages that you enjoy. Obviously, the sugar-laden beverages must stop. They contribute a large amount of unnecessary dietary energy. If you have not already done so, switching to non-calorie beverages is a first step. Avoid so-called light beverages. Light drinks still contain carbohydrate calories, simply less than another product.

Many are critical of the use of diet beverages, particularly because of the sweetener aspartame. This criticism is valid, but people react differently to the use of aspartame, and sugar is the greater health danger.

Carbonated beverages, by themselves, are an issue for some. For those troubled by reflux or heartburn, both the acid and the gas in these beverages may worsen their problems. If this is not the case, but you wish to avoid aspartame, club soda or seltzer may be a reasonable substitute. You can add non-calorie flavorings and sweeteners that you trust.

Caffeine has been portrayed either as a health villain or as completely harmless. Coffee, which contains caffeine, has been in human use for about a thousand years. Originating in Africa and Middle East, it reached Europe about 500 years ago. It is a mild drug that increases alertness. In moderate use, it is safe for the average person. Scientific reviews have concluded that between three and five cups a day are safe for most people. Unfortunately, the scientific definition is often confused because of changing patterns of coffee consumption. The accepted definition of a cup of coffee in the United States is usually about five and two thirds fluid ounces (about 167 ml.) and it is somewhat less in Europe. Today, coffee mugs and restaurant servings typically are twelve, sixteen, and even twenty ounces. Therefore, using today's common cup size, safe and moderate caffeine use may be limited to two of these larger cups of coffee each day.

Caffeine is closely related to theophylline, found in tea and theobromine, found in chocolate. Caffeine is actually sold as a drug in certain headache medications and theophylline is a drug found in some asthma medications. They're both useful drugs in those circumstances. At higher doses, this mild drug can take on more unpleasant effects. It may cause anxiety, and it may increase heart rate and blood pressure. In older men with prostate problems it can cause urinary difficulty. Caffeine is also a mild diuretic, which increases urine production. Although you are taking in more fluid by drinking these beverages, you may not become better hydrated, since you lose more in urination.

At very high doses caffeine also suppresses the appetite. At one time, the "secret" ingredient in many over-the-counter diet pills was simply extremely concentrated caffeine. These were eventually pulled from the market because of the complications they caused. At extremely high doses, it can mimic the side-effects of cocaine or amphetamine.

This dietary plan is neither for nor against caffeine use. Most people will continue to enjoy their morning coffee without change. In fact, a teaspoon of real cream in that coffee has helped many stay on diet. The purpose of this discussion is to give you a better understanding, so that you can make your own informed choices.

One caution is that suddenly stopping caffeine use can be a problem. People who use high amounts of coffee or caffeinated soft-drinks will feel fatigue, depressed, and suffer severe headaches, if they suddenly stop. Normally, this clears up in about a week. If the source of your caffeine is coffee, switching to decaffeinated coffee does not eliminate all of your caffeine. Decaffeinated products contain reduced caffeine, but they are not totally caffeine-free. On the other hand, soft-drinks have no natural caffeine until it has been added, so switching to caffeine-free soda definitely eliminates that source of caffeine.

Many beverage alternatives exist. Some people

like the taste of a drop or two of lemon or lime juice in a glass of ordinary water, or even a drop of malt or cider vinegar. Caffeine-free herbal teas, as well as Asian barley tea, can be served either hot or cold. Fruit-flavored syrups popular in coffee houses are available in sugar-free varieties and can be added to many drinks, including club soda.

Is it necessary to have beverages at all? Yes, drinking water with your meal will definitely reduce the amount that you eat. Drinking water shortly before your meal may help, too. The old standby, eight glasses of water each day, is a myth without scientific basis. In reality, you may need more or less depending upon your individual needs. The easiest gauge is observing your urine. If you are taking in too much fluid, your urine may become extremely pale and look like water. On the other hand, if you are dehydrated and not receiving enough daily fluid, your urine output will drop and its color will darken.

The recipes that follow provide a few extra choices for your beverage selection.

Beverages

Hot Chocolate

Serves 1

Use this recipe when you need a chocolate lift or to warm yourself on a dreary winter day. You also may refrigerate it to serve cold, either by itself or mixed with club soda.

Ingredients	_Amount_
100% cocoa powder	1 teaspoon
Cream	1 tablespoon
Liquid non-calorie sweetener	To taste
Hot water	To fill cup

Instructions: Pour hot to boiling water over cocoa powder and stir until dissolved. Add cream, sweeten to taste, and stir.

Energy	65 calories
Fat	6 grams
Protein	½ gram
Carbohydrate	1 gram

Lemonade or Limeade
Serves 1

At home, this is a refreshing and inexpensive beverage, providing a healthier alternative to carbonated soft drinks.

Eating out, the only non-alcohol beverage choices are often either water or something containing either sugar or caffeine. Fight back, by simply asking for a slice of lemon or lime in your water. That way, it is free of both sugar and caffeine, as well as free-of-charge.

Ingredients	Amount
Water	1 glass
Lemon or lime	1 slice or juice to taste
Non-calorie sweetener	To taste

Instructions: At home, you may wish to use concentrated lemon or lime juice, if you do not have a fresh lemon or lime available. Liquid sweetener is preferable to powdered.

When eating out, ask for a slice of lemon or lime in your water. Squeeze the lemon into you glass and use non-calorie sweetener to taste.

Tip the waitress a little more for her trouble; you still save money compared to a soft drink.

Energy	0 calories
Fat	0 grams
Protein	0 grams
Carbohydrate	0 grams

Real Cream Soda

Serves 1

Whether you want to increase the proportion of fat in a particular meal or just have a delicious treat, try this real cream soda. This delicious beverage may remind you of an old-fashioned ice cream float.

Ingredients	*Amount*
Cream	1 tablespoon
Ice cubes	1 or 2, to taste
Diet soda in a flavor such as cream, root beer, cola, or orange.	Enough to fill glass

Instructions: Place ice in the glass first, then add the cream. Next, slowly pour in the soda. Stir briefly, if needed, as it froths. Drink up and enjoy.

Hint: *Rather than use a flavored diet soda, try it with a small amount of sugar-free flavored syrup, filling the glass with either unflavored seltzer or club soda. Sugar-free syrups are often sold in coffee-houses, where they are used for flavored coffees and Italian sodas. Some groceries and specialty food shops also carry them, often in the coffee section. Pick flavors you like, but be careful to get the sugar-free variety.*

Energy	54 calories
Fat	6 grams
Protein	0 grams
Carbohydrate	0 grams

Chapter 6

Treats

Being on a diet should not mean that you give up desserts or treats. Just remember that these are special foods and reserve some of them for special occasions. In this area in particular, I would like to thank my patients and my readers for their many ideas and contributions.

There are some special treats commercially available that are acceptable. A few low-carbohydrate ice cream treats and many sugar-free candies can meet the requirements of this dietary plan. However, many of these are loaded with sugar alcohol. Used moderately, this is fine, but people react individually. Do not forget that some individuals will develop gas, bloating, and diarrhea even at small levels of sugar alcohol.

The best choices are often those treats you make yourself. Try some of them!

Treats

Brownies

Serves 4

Satisfy your sweet tooth.

Ingredients	*Amount*
Butter	2 tablespoons
Cocoa powder	2 tablespoons
Vanilla	Splash
Egg	1
Liquid sweetener	6 drops
Baking powder	½ teaspoon
Splenda®	1 teaspoon
Oil	1 tablespoon
Almond flour	2 tablespoons

Instructions: Melt butter. Mix all ingredients, stirring well. Pour into a small (about 5" by 5") baking dish or 4 cupcake papers in a tin. Bake at 350° for 10 minutes. Allow to cool and serve.

Almond flour is made from ground almonds. It is available in many natural food stores and in some supermarkets.

Energy	**134**	**calories**
Fat	**13**	**grams**
Protein	**3**	**grams**
Carbohydrate	**1**	**grams**

Cheese Crisps

Serves 1

Tasty snack or side dish.

Ingredients	Amount
Fresh grated parmesan cheese	2 tablespoons
Fresh grated Asiago cheese	2 tablespoons
Oregano or basil	Optional, to taste

Instructions: Mix cheeses and optional herbs. Spoon 4 small mounds of about 1 tablespoon each on a non-stick cookie sheet. Bake at 425° for 8 to 10 minutes until brown and crisp. Remove immediately, shape if desired. Allow to cool and serve.

.

Energy	97	**calories**
Fat	11	**grams**
Protein	8	**grams**
Carbohydrate	1	**grams**

Cheesecake

Serves 16

A special treat for holidays and special occasions.

<u>Ingredients</u>	<u>Amount</u>
Crust	
Ground hazelnuts	⅔ cup
Almond flour	¾ cup
Splenda®	½ cup
Liquid non-calorie sweetener	1 tablespoon
Butter	¼ cup
Filling	
Cream Cheese	24 ounces
Cream	1 cup
Eggs	4
Splenda®	¾ cup
Liquid non-calorie sweetener	1 tablespoon
Vanilla extract	1 teaspoon

Instructions: Preheat oven to 350 F. Line the bottom of a 10 inch diameter springform pan with an appropriate cardboard or parchment paper liner on the bottom to make removal easier. Cover the outside of the springform pan with a single sheet of aluminum foil to make it waterproof on the bottom and sides.

Mix the crust ingredients together by hand. Pack it firmly and evenly in the bottom of the springform pan. Start the filling by first mixing Splenda® and cream cheese in a large bowl. Now add the eggs, one at a time, while you continue to mix. Finally, mix the cream, vanilla, and liquid sweetener.

(continued on the next page)

Pour your filling mixture into the springform pan. Find a large baking pan that the springform pan can fit into. Now, pour about 2 cups of water in the large outside pan and carefully set the springform pan into the larger pan. The water should come partially up the side of the springform pan. You have just created a *bain marie,* which will help your cheesecake cook in a way that will reduce cracking.

Put these into your oven and bake at 350° for 1 hour. Turn off after 1 hour but leave in the oven with the door open for another hour. Now, remove the springform pan from the *bain marie.*

You may wish to gently run a knife around the outside of the cheesecake at this time. Allow the cheesecake to cool in your refrigerator for another hour or more before serving. When serving, rinse or dip your serving knife in hot water to minimize sticking.

Almond flour is made from ground almonds. It is available in many natural food stores and in some supermarkets.

Energy	353	calories
Fat	35	grams
Protein	7	grams
Carbohydrate	1	grams

Treats

Chocolate Coconut Candy
Serves 30

Makes a large batch of candy to freeze or share.

Ingredient	Amount
Eggs	4
Splenda® sweetener	1½ cups
Shredded unsweetened coconut	3 cups
Unsweetened baking chocolate	2 one-ounce squares
Coconut extract flavoring	1 teaspoon

Instructions: Separate egg whites. Discard the yolks or use them for another recipe. Beat the whites with a mixer until they increase in volume and begin to stiffen. Add coconut extract then slowly add Splenda® while continuing to beat until stiff. Now, mix in shredded coconut. Use a greased or parchment lined cookie sheet and spoon out into 30 small mounds, shaping into a smooth shape. Bake about 12 minutes in a preheated oven at 325^0. Allow them to cool briefly before transferring to a cooling rack for further cooling.

Now, carefully melt the baking chocolate, using a microwave or double boiler. Decorate the coconut mounds with the melted chocolate and allow to cool completely before serving or freezing.

Caution: Do not overdo the Splenda®. If possible, substitute some liquid sweetener.

Energy	**52 calories**
Fat	**4 grams**
Protein	**2 grams**
Carbohydrate	**2 grams**

Toasted Cinnamon Glazed Nuts

32 Servings of ½ ounce or about 10 nuts

When you bake these, you may recall the aroma coming from a nut shop in a mall around holiday time. You may substitute other nuts for the almonds.

Ingredients	*Amount*
Raw almonds	1 pound
Egg white	1
Water	1 teaspoon
Splenda®	1 cup
Cinnamon	1 tablespoon
Salt	1 teaspoon
Cocoa powder	1 teaspoon *(optional)*

Instructions: Using an electric mixer, beat the egg white and water until frothy. In another bowl, mix Splenda®, cinnamon, and salt. Add nuts to the egg mixture. Stir until coated with the egg, then pour in the powder mixture and stir again, until all the nuts have been evenly coated. Spread the nuts evenly on a cookie sheet that has been greased or lined with parchment paper. Bake at 250^0 (or lower in a convection oven) for 1 hour, stirring every 15 minutes. Allow the nuts to cool completely before bagging or they may not be crunchy!

Use small snack bags to separate individual portions and be careful to not overdo portions.

Caution: Do not overdo the Splenda®. If possible, substitute some liquid sweetener.

Energy	83 calories
Fat	7 grams
Protein	3 grams
Carbohydrate	2 grams

Cream Cheese Fudge

Serves 18

Make this for a large group or freeze individual servings.

Ingredients	*Amount*	
Sugar-free chocolate sauce	4	tablespoons
Cream cheese	16	ounces
Splenda®	3	teaspoons
Vanilla	¼	teaspoon

Instructions: Combine all ingredients completely. Place mixture in a 9 by 6 inch pan lined with aluminum foil and spread evenly. Cover with plastic wrap and chill overnight. Cut into 18 pieces before serving.

If you wish, add crushed nuts to the mixture before chilling. Remember to add these nuts to the nutritional values.

Energy	88	**calories**
Fat	9	**grams**
Protein	2	**grams**
Carbohydrate	1	**grams**

Creamy Chocolate Dessert
Serves 1

This simple recipe provides a proportioned balance of energy, while allowing you to have a chocolate treat. It is a great addition to a light meal.

Ingredients	*Amount*
Sour cream	2 tablespoons
Cocoa powder	1 teaspoon
Liquid non-calorie sweetener	to taste

Instructions: Stir together until the chocolate is evenly distributed. Taste and stir in extra sweetener, as needed.

Energy	**62**	**calories**
Fat	**6**	**grams**
Protein	**1**	**grams**
Carbohydrate	**1**	**grams**

Flaxseed Bread

Serves 24

Freeze portions that will not be used within 2 days.

<u>Ingredients</u>	<u>Amount</u>
Flaxseed meal (golden)	2 cups
Baking powder	1 tablespoon
Liquid non-calorie sweetener	¾ teaspoon
Eggs	4
Water	½ cup
Olive oil	⅓ cup

Instructions: Preheat oven to 350^0. Prepare an 8 by 12 inch pan with oiled parchment paper to prevent sticking. Mix dry ingredients well. Beat eggs, mix wet ingredients together, then add wet to dry, and combine well. Let batter set for 3 minutes to thicken, then pour into pan and spread it evenly. Bake for about 20 minutes, until it springs back when you touch the top and is visibly brown. Cut into 2 by 2 inch portions. You may split these and use them for sandwiches.

Golden flaxseed is tastier than the dark variety. You may wish to mix both or grind your own meal from less expensive whole flaxseed. These are available in natural food stores and some supermarkets. Store flaxseed meal tightly closed in the refrigerator to prevent rancidity.

Hint: Add sugar-free imitation honey to recipe for flavor. Check www.HoneyTreeHoney.com to find where to buy it.

Energy	113	**calories**
Fat	10	**grams**
Protein	5	**grams**
Carbohydrate	0	**grams**

Peanut Butter Cookies

Serves 20

Light and tasty

Ingredients	Amount
Natural peanut butter	1 cup
Splenda	1 cup
Egg	1
Real vanilla extract	1 teaspoon, *to taste*

Instructions: Separate the egg, beat the white until fluffy. Mix other ingredients together. Fold egg white into the rest of the mixture. Using a parchment lined or pre-greased cookie sheet, place 20 cookies of about a tablespoon each and flatten slightly. Bake at 350° for 8 to 10 minutes.

Caution: Do not overdo the Splenda®. If possible, substitute some liquid sweetener.

Energy	85	calories
Fat	6	grams
Protein	3	grams
Carbohydrate	1	grams

Pumpkin Pie

Serves 8

A Thanksgiving treat.

Ingredient	Amount
Cream cheese	8 ounce package
Splenda®	1 cup
Eggs	3
Cream	¾ cup
Pumpkin pie filling	1 15 ounce can
Almond extract	1 teaspoon
Pumpkin pie spice	1 tablespoon
Vanilla extract	1 teaspoon
Salt	½ teaspoon

Instructions: Prepare bottom layer by mixing cream cheese, ¼ cup Splenda®, almond extract, and 1 egg. Spoon mixture into a greased 8 by 8 inch baking pan.

Prepare the second layer by separating the whites of the remaining 2 eggs and beating the whites until fluffy. Now, mix in the yolks and remaining ingredients. Pour this over the first layer.

Bake for 15 minutes in an oven preheated to 400°, then lower the oven temperature to 325° and bake for an additional 45 minutes. Remove from the oven and cool. Chill in refrigerator before serving.

Caution: Do not overdo the Splenda®. If possible, substitute some liquid sweetener.

Energy	**236**	**calories**
Fat	**20**	**grams**
Protein	**4**	**grams**
Carbohydrate	**5**	**grams**

Real Whipped Cream
Serves 1

A delicious way to add fat to balance your meal.
Works well during initiation to this diet.

Ingredient	Amount
Cream	2 tablespoons
Liquid non-calorie sweetener	To taste.

Instructions: Use a chilled glass bowl and whip the cream until stiff with an electric mixer, adding the liquid sweetener as you mix.

You may wish to serve this over sugar-free Jell-O®. If so, do not use the prepared variety. Flavors labeled "5 calories per serving" are preferred. Prepare this in advance following the label instructions.

	Alone	With Jell-O®	
Energy	90	95	calories
Fat	10	10	grams
Protein	0	1	grams
Carbohydrate	0	0	grams

Rhubarb Custard
Serves 6

May be made with fresh or frozen rhubarb.

Ingredients	Amount
Eggs	3
Water	½ cup
Cream	1 cup
Splenda®	1 ½ cups
Butter	4 tablespoons
Vanilla extract	2 teaspoons
Orange zest	½ teaspoon
Rhubarb (finely chopped)	2 ½ cups

Instructions: Defrost rhubarb, if frozen. Combine rhubarb and ½ cup Splenda® and microwave on high for 1 minute.

In a different bowl, melt butter and mix all remaining ingredients for the custard mix.

Put the rhubarb mixture into 6 ramekins (small glass baking dishes) or a lined cupcake tin. Cover with the custard mix.

Bake at 275° for 35 to 40 minutes. Remove from oven and allow to cool. Chill in refrigerator before serving.

Caution: Do not overdo the Splenda®. If possible, substitute some liquid sweetener.

Energy	**256**	**calories**
Fat	**25**	**grams**
Protein	**4**	**grams**
Carbohydrate	**3**	**grams**

Rhubarb Dessert

Serves 12

Another great rhubarb recipe. Use fresh or frozen rhubarb.

Ingredients	*Amount*
Rhubarb (finely chopped)	2 cups
Cream cheese (softened)	8 ounces
Eggs	5
Cream	½ cup
White vinegar	1 teaspoon
Cinnamon	2 teaspoons
Vanilla	1 teaspoon
Splenda®	1 ⅔ cups

Instructions: Allow frozen rhubarb to thaw and cream cheese to soften at room temperature. Heat the rhubarb with 1 cup of Splenda® in a small saucepan over low heat until the Splenda® is dissolved and the rhubarb has softened.

Using an electric mixer, combine all the remaining ingredients in a bowl, then fold in the rhubarb mixture. Pour into a greased 8 by 8 inch pan and bake at 325° for about 45 minutes. The center should spring back when touched. Allow to cool. May be served at room temperature or chilled.

Caution: Do not overdo the Splenda®. If possible, substitute some liquid sweetener.

Energy	**127**	**calories**
Fat	**11**	**grams**
Protein	**4**	**grams**
Carbohydrate	**2**	**grams**

Sesame Crackers

Serves 12

Based upon 2 crackers per serving.

Ingredients	_Amount_
Almond meal	1 cup
Sesame seeds	¼ cup
Grated parmesan cheese	4 ounces
Prepared mustard	2 teaspoons
Egg	1
Garlic powder	1 teaspoon
Salt	¼ teaspoon

Instructions: Separate egg and discard yolk. Combine all ingredients, using a food processor until ingredients cling together in a ball. Roll dough by hand, into a cylinder about 1½ inches in diameter. Slice cylinder with a knife, into 24 pieces, about 3 slices to an inch.

Place the slices on a baking sheet covered with parchment paper and flatten so that they are about 2 inches in diameter. Bake in an oven preheated to 325° for about 14 to 18 minutes, removing when they begin to brown. Allow crackers to cool and store in an airtight container.

Almond meal is made from ground almonds, but it is a little coarser than almond flour. It is available in many natural food stores and in some supermarkets. You may substitute almond flour if almond meal is not available.

Energy	106	**calories**
Fat	6	**grams**
Protein	9	**grams**
Carbohydrate	5	**grams**

Chapter 7

Condiments

Condiments include sauces, spices, and relishes used to season food. Unfortunately, many of the commercially available condiments contain either sugar or MSG. The good news is that it is easy to make your own condiments. The recipes in this chapter are quick, easy, and delicious. Many of them go well with a variety of foods.

Condiments

Avocado Dressing
Serves 16

Based upon a serving size of about 2 tablespoons.

Ingredients	Amount
Avocado	1 (large)
Lemon juice	2 tablespoons
Mayonnaise	1 cup
Sour cream	½ cup
Chipotle sauce	1 teaspoon *(to taste)*
Onion, chopped	⅓ cup *(to taste)*
Garlic , minced	2 cloves *(to taste)*
Salt	1 teaspoon *(to taste)*
Cayenne pepper	dash *(to taste)*

Instructions: You may wish to vary or reduce quantities of onions, garlic, and spices to suit your taste. Use a blender or food processor to blend all ingredients together. Chill before serving.

Energy	137 calories
Fat	15 grams
Protein	1 grams
Carbohydrate	2 grams

Barbecue and Meat Sauce

Serves 1

This is a terrific sauce for cooking meat and as a base for other sauces. It is almost calorie-free and can be made in advance and stored. The key ingredient is chipotle sauce, a thick brown sauce made from smoked chili peppers. It can be found in the Mexican food section of many supermarkets and specialty stores.

Ingredients	*Amount*
Chipotle sauce	All quantities to taste
Ground cinnamon	All quantities to taste
Non-calorie liquid sweetener	All quantities to taste
Fresh or bottled lemon juice	All quantities to taste

Instructions: Mix ingredients together until completely blended. Quantities can be varied to your taste. Brush on meat or poultry before cooking. May also be used at the table, in place of commercial steak sauce.

Energy	0	calories
Fat	0	grams
Protein	0	grams
Carbohydrate	0	grams

Basil Garlic Mayonnaise
Serves 16

Serving size about 1 tablespoon for this rich pesto-like sauce.

Ingredients	*Amount*
Fresh basil	1 cup, loosely packed
Garlic	1 clove *(to taste)*
Salt	¼ teaspoon *(to taste)*
Cayenne pepper	⅛ teaspoon *(to taste)*
Mayonnaise	¾ cup

Instructions: You may wish to vary amounts of spices according to your preference. Using a food processor, pulse-chop all ingredients except the mayonnaise until the basil is finely chopped. Add the mayonnaise and continue mixing until smooth. Chill in refrigerator for at least an hour to let the flavors fully blend and develop.

Energy	75 calories
Fat	9 grams
Protein	0 grams
Carbohydrate	0 grams

Chunky Bleu or Feta Cheese Dressing

Serves 14

Use a two tablespoon serving either as a salad dressing, a sauce to top meat, fish, and vegetables, or as a dip. If your meals are out of balance, using this as a topping is a delicious way to add fat.

<u>Ingredients</u>	<u>Amount</u>
Crumbled bleu or feta cheese*	¼ cup
Mayonnaise	½ cup
Sour cream	1 cup
Hot sauce *(optional)*	A few drops, to taste

Instructions: Mix ingredients. Refrigerate unused portion.

Hint: The small amount of carbohydrate is based upon using cheese that is pre-crumbled. However, if you use blocks of cheese and crumble it yourself, you will reduce this.

Pre-crumbled and pre-grated cheeses are powdered with a light coating of starch, to prevent them from sticking together after packaging.

Energy	100	**calories**
Fat	11	**grams**
Protein	1	**gram**
Carbohydrate	1	**gram**

Condiments

Creamy Curry Sauce

Serves 1

A single tablespoon of this simple sauce is a great way to balance the proportion of fat in meals, while adding taste. It goes well when used as a topping on many foods.

Try it on lightly steamed asparagus.

Ingredients	*Amount*
Mayonnaise	1 tablespoon
Curry Powder	½ teaspoon, *to taste*

Instructions: Mix the curry powder and mayonnaise thoroughly. Allow to stand a few minutes before using.

If larger amounts are mixed, be sure to refrigerate any unused portion.

Energy	108	calories
Fat	12	grams
Protein	0	grams
Carbohydrate	0	grams

Creamy Dill Dip
Serves 16

Use a tablespoon for a snack, party dip or topping.

<u>Ingredients</u>	<u>Amount</u>
Sour cream	½ Cup
Mayonnaise	½ Cup
Dried onion flakes	½ tablespoon, *to taste*
Dry dill weeds	½ tablespoon, *to taste*
Salt	¼ teaspoon, *to taste*
Pepper	dash, *to taste*

Instructions: Mix all ingredients. Chill in refrigerator before serving.

Energy	**66 calories**
Fat	**7 grams**
Protein	**0 grams**
Carbohydrate	**1 grams**

Condiments

Creamy Salsa Salad Dressing and Dip
SERVES 14

Use 2 tablespoons as a dip or a dressing.

Ingredients	Amount
Sour Cream	1 cup
Mayonnaise	¼ cup
Herdez® Salsa	½ cup
Salsa Seasoning*	2 teaspoons, *to taste*

Instructions: Mix all ingredients and allow flavors to blend while chilling in refrigerator.

* such as Tastefully Simple® Simply Salsa Mix™.

Look for ingredients in the Latin food section of your local market. Be sure the products you find are free of sugar and MSG.

Energy	75	**calories**
Fat	7	**grams**
Protein	1	**grams**
Carbohydrate	2	**grams**

Herb Seasoning

Serves 8

You may wish to use a teaspoon of this homemade
seasoning mix instead of commercial mixes.

Ingredients	**Amount**
Dill weed	2 tablespoons
Onion powder	2 Tablespoons, (*optional*)
Oregano	1 teaspoon
Dried lemon peel	½ teaspoon
Salt and pepper	dash

Instructions: Use a small coffee or spice mill to grind the
dried lemon peel to powder. Mix all ingredients well and save
in an appropriate container.

Hint: Skip the onion powder to eliminate carbohydrate content.

Energy	4 calories
Fat	0 grams
Protein	0 grams
Carbohydrate	1 grams

Condiments

Olive Dip

Serves 14

Use a 2 tablespoon serving with cauliflower, broccoli, celery or pork rinds for a party dip.

Ingredients	_Amount_	
Sour Cream	4	tablespoons
Mayonnaise	2	tablespoons
Minced black olives	¼	small *(4½ ounce)* can
Minced onion	3	tablespoons
Minced tomatoes	3	tablespoons
Minced fresh cilantro	2	tablespoons
Lime juice	2	teaspoons
Minced garlic	½	cloves
Hot sauce	1	teaspoon, *(to taste)*

Instructions: Mince ingredients, as needed, then combine. Chill in the refrigerator to allow flavors to mix before serving.

Energy	47	**calories**
Fat	5	**grams**
Protein	0	**grams**
Carbohydrate	1	**grams**

Tartar Sauce

Serves 10

Use a tablespoon of this traditional sauce to balance fat content serving when lighter-color high-protein fish.

Ingredients	**Amount**
Mayonnaise	½ cup
Chopped onion	1 tablespoon
Lemon juice	1 tablespoon
Dill weed	½ teaspoon
Mustard	½ teaspoon powder (or prepared)
Paprika	¼ teaspoon
Black pepper	¼ teaspoon

Instructions: Mix all ingredients together, refrigerate, and chill before serving.

Hint: Add unsweetened dill pickle relish, if desired.

Energy	79 calories
Fat	9 grams
Protein	0 grams
Carbohydrate	0 grams

Appendix A

Measurement Equivalents
Approximate

Volume

1 teaspoon	5 milliliter
1 tablespoon	3 teaspoons
1 tablespoon	15 milliliter
16 tablespoons	1 cup
1 cup	240 milliliter
¼ cup	60 milliliter
½ cup	120 milliliter
¾ cup	180 milliliter

Note: Volume measures refer to U.S. units, not Imperial units.

Weight

1 ounce	28 grams
1 pound	454 grams

Oven temperature

275°F	135°C	Gas Mark 1
300°F	150°C	Gas Mark 2
325°F	165°C	Gas Mark 3
350°F	180°C	Gas Mark 4
375°F	195°C	Gas Mark 5

Liquid Sweetener

Amounts are for sweetener where 6 drops (about 2 ml.) are equal to 1 teaspoon (5 ml.) sugar. Adjust for other strength sweeteners.

Appendix B

Recipe Worksheets

These worksheets are for developing your own recipes or checking recipes you find elsewhere. As you list each ingredient and amount, fill in the grams for fat, protein, and carbohydrate. Total these amounts, then divide these results by the number of servings to determine grams per serving.

Recipe Worksheet

Recipe for _____

Number of servings _____

Ingredient & Amount	F gm 9	P gm 4	C gm 4	calories
1				
2				
3				
4				
5				
6				
7				
8				
9				
10				
Totals per recipe add columns	grams	grams	grams	calories

Divide the above line by the number of servings in this recipe.

Amounts per Serving	grams	grams	grams	calories

Cooking instructions & comments:

Appendix B

Recipe Worksheet

Recipe for _____

Number of servings _____

Ingredient & Amount	F gm 9	P gm 4	C gm 4	calories
1				
2				
3				
4				
5				
6				
7				
8				
9				
10				
Totals per recipe *add columns*	grams	grams	grams	calories

Divide the above line by the number of servings in this recipe.

Amounts per Serving	grams	grams	grams	calories

Cooking instructions & comments:

Appendix B

Recipe Worksheet

Recipe for _____

Number of servings _____

Ingredient & Amount	F gm 9	P gm 4	C gm 4	calories
1				
2				
3				
4				
5				
6				
7				
8				
9				
10				
Totals per recipe *add columns*	grams	grams	grams	calories

Divide the above line by the number of servings in this recipe.

Amounts per Serving	grams	grams	grams	calories

Cooking instructions & comments:

Appendix B

Recipe Worksheet

Recipe for _____

Number of servings _____

Ingredient & Amount	F gm 9	P gm 4	C gm 4	calories
1				
2				
3				
4				
5				
6				
7				
8				
9				
10				
Totals per recipe *add columns*	grams	grams	grams	calories

Divide the above line by the number of servings in this recipe.

Amounts per Serving	grams	grams	grams	calories

Cooking instructions & comments:

Appendix B

Recipe Worksheet

Recipe for _____

Number of servings _____

Ingredient & Amount	F gm **9**	P gm **4**	C gm **4**	calories
1				
2				
3				
4				
5				
6				
7				
8				
9				
10				
Totals per recipe *add columns*	grams	grams	grams	calories

Divide the above line by the number of servings in this recipe.

Amounts per Serving	grams	grams	grams	calories

Cooking instructions & comments:

Recipe Worksheet

Recipe for _____

Number of servings _____

Ingredient & Amount	**F** gm *9*	**P** gm *4*	**C** gm *4*	calories
1				
2				
3				
4				
5				
6				
7				
8				
9				
10				
Totals per recipe *add columns*	grams	grams	grams	calories

Divide the above line by the number of servings in this recipe.

Amounts per Serving				
	grams	grams	grams	calories

Cooking instructions & comments:

152

Appendix C

Keeping A Diary

People following a dietary plan are most likely to succeed when they record their food intake, test readings their plan calls for, and their weight progress. A daily diary sheet allows you to do this easily. If you record this information, review it at the end of the day, and you will be able to easily determine how close you are to your plan.

This is how one woman used her daily diary:

- She recorded the date and day .
- She started the day recording her weight and test results. Because she is diabetic, these included sugar.
- After meals, she subtracted her grams from the 60/40/10 reminders at the top of the columns, so that she could see how much she had left to work with during the day.
- Her urine test for ketosis was large in the morning but slightly less during the active day, when her body was burning ketones as fast as it was supplying them.
- Her weight varied during the day but should be less the following day.

- At the end of the day, she totaled up 64/39/7, reasonably close to her goal. She could multiply the grams to calculate her total calories.

As her glucose is well-controlled while her weight falls, she knows what she has done and what works best for her.

Diaries are available at
www.HippocraticDiet.com

Date: July 1			This is day 38 of my diet.			
New Hippocratic Diet® Daily Diary						
Time	Food Item or Test or Weight	Test Results	FAT grams 60 x9	PROTEIN grams 40 x4	CARBS grams 10 x4	calories (optional)
6:30	weight	237 1/2				
"	glucose	97				
"	ketosis	large				
7:15	Coffee + tbs. cream		5	-	-	
"	omelet		11 (44)	6 (36)	1 (9)	
9:15	glucose	108				
10:30	Coffee + tbs. cream		5	-	-	
12:45	Salad, blue cheese		6	2	4	
"	Cream soda		5 (28)	- (34)	- (5)	
2:45	glucose	109				
6 pm	ketosis	moderate				
"	weight	238				
6:30	3 oz salmon/oil		11	20	-	
"	4 Asparagus		-	1	2	
"	Curry sauce		11	-	-	
"	Iced tea		- (6)	- (13)	- (3)	
8:30	glucose	110				
9 pm	Munster cheese x2		10	12	-	
Daily Totals add columns			64 (576) grams	39 (156) grams	7 (28) grams	780 calories
Special events and comments						
Felt great during the day, had a high energy level. Had 2 slices of cheese as a snack at night.						

Index

A

Acesulfame, 11
Addiction: The High-Low Trap, 167
Africa, origin of coffee, 111
African slaves, and sugar, 7
Alertness from coffee, 111
Alfredo sauce, 6, 62
Alfredo Sauce Recipe, 62
ALS, food additives, 11
American Board of Addiction Medicine, 168
American College of Preventive Medicine, 168
Ancient India, sugar and disease in, 7
Ancient Persia, sugar and disease in, 7
Anxiety, from coffee, 111
increases heart rate and blood pressure, 111
Artificial sweeteners, 8-9
Asian restaurant, appetizers at, 17
Asparagus, 25, 87, 91, 105
Asparagus Soup Recipe, 105
Chilled Marinated Asparagus Recipe, 91
Aspartame, 10, 110
Asthma medication, with theophylline, 111
Author information, 168
Autism from food additives, 11
Avocado, 4, 79
Avocado Dressing, 134
Avocado, Grilled Recipe, 57

B

Bacteria and sugar alcohols, 11
Baked Catfish Recipe, 42
Balsamic vinegar, 78
Barbecue and Meat Sauce Recipe, 135
Barbecue sauce, 66, 134
Basil Garlic Dressing, 136
Beans, 79
Beef,
    Citrus Steak, 18
    Flank Steak, 19
    Mexican Beef, 21
    Mexican Burgers, 22
    Mexican Cubed Steak, 23
Beer in ancient Mesopotamia, 109
Beets, 87
Beverages, 109
    Hot Chocolate Recipe, 114
    Lemonade, 115
    Limeade, 116
    Real Cream Soda, 117
Bible, on wine, 109
Board-certified in,
    Addiction Medicine, 168
    Preventive Medicine and Public Health, 168
Bottled sauces, with sugar and MSG, 14
Bottled water, 110
Brand names, 7
Bread, Flaxseed, 126
Breading substitutes, 68

Index

Index

Index

Index

Poultry, 68
  Chicken Baked Recipe, 68
  Chicken Mole Recipe, 69
  Chicken with Creamy
    Mustard Sauce Recipe, 71
  Chicken with Lemon Recipe,
    75
  Chicken Salad Recipe, 70
  Hearty Chicken Stew Recipe,
    73-74
  Spicy Chicken Wings Recipe,
    76
  Spicy Lime Chicken Recipe,
    77
  turkey, 68
Powdered soup, 103
Pre-crumbled cheese, 137
Pregnant women, 6
Pre-grated cheese, 137
Preventive Medicine
  Associates, 152
Prostate problems, 111-12
Pumpkin Pie Recipe, 128

Q

Quiche Recipe, 40
Quick Salmon and Cream
  Recipe, 48

R

Rare spice, sugar as, 7
Raw eggs, dangerous, 35
Real Cream Soda, 117
Real mayonnaise, 14, 78-79
Real Whipped Cream Recipe,
  129
Recipe sharing, 16
Recipe Worksheet, 147
Red dye, 15
Red peppers
  Roasted Red Pepper Soup
    Recipe, 108

Reflux, and carbonated
  beverages, 110-11
Rhubarb Custard Recipe, 130
Rhubarb Dessert Recipe, 131
Ricotta Cheese Soufflé, 30
Roasted Red Pepper Recipe,
  108
Russian dressing, 79

S

Saccharin, 8-9
Safe foods, myth, 6
Salad dressings, 78-79
Salads, 78-80
  chef's salad, 79-80
  Cobb salad, 79
  Egg. Bacon, and Avocado
    Recipe, 81
Salmon, dark varieties, 41
  eat twice per week, 45
Salt, 15
Salt substitute, 15, 16
Salted butter, 14
Sardines, 41, 79
Sauces, 135, 138, 143
  Barbecue And Meat Sauce
    Recipe, 135
  Tartar Sauce Recipe, 143
Sausage-Stuffed Jalapenos
  Recipe, 84
Seafood Salad Recipe, 49
Seltzer, 111
Sesame Crackers Recipe, 132
Sesame oil, 14, 79
Shirakiku®, 60
Shirataki noodles, 59-60, 64
Shortening, avoid, 14
Shrimp, 41
  Shrimp and Spinach Recipe,
    50
  Shrimp in Creamy Mustard
    Sauce Recipe, 51

Index

Other Books by Dr. Cohen

Diabetes Recovery:
Reversing Diabetes with the
New Hippocratic Diet®
Center for Health Information, 2010
ISBN 978-0-9820111-0-2

Doctor Cohen's New Hippocratic Diet® Guide:
How to Really Lose Weight and Beat the
Obesity Epidemic
Center for Health Information, 2008
ISBN 978-0-9820111-9-5

Addiction: The High-Low Trap
Health Press, 1995
ISBN 0-929173-10-4

*To order these
or for additional copies of this book,
go to*

www.CenterForHealthInformation.com

About the Author

Irving Cohen, M.D., M.P.H. is a physician who has dedicated his medical career to the prevention of disease, focusing on early detection and interventions to prevent later more serious diseases. He directs Preventive Medicine Associates and serves as a volunteer physician serving the uninsured at the Marian Clinic of the Little Sisters of Charity. He and his wife, Lauren, have resided in Kansas for almost twenty years.

Earlier, he had retired but became interested in the emerging epidemics of overweight, obesity, and diabetes. His research prompted his return to practice.

Dr. Cohen has served in private practice and government service, in public health and clinical medicine. He has served as Deputy Director of the New York State Research Institute on Addiction. He held faculty appointments at the State University of New York at Buffalo, School of Medicine, in both the Departments of Medicine as well as Social and Preventive Medicine. He has held faculty appointments at the University of Kansas, School of Medicine in the Department of the History of Medicine as well as the Department of Preventive Medicine. He held a faculty appointment at the Karl Menninger School of Psychiatry and Mental Health Sciences.

Dr. Cohen received his training in Preventive Medicine and Public Health at the Johns Hopkins University, Bloomberg School of Public Health in Baltimore, Maryland. He served as Chief Resident of Preventive Medicine at that institution. Dr. Cohen is a Fellow of the American College of Preventive Medicine. He is Board-Certified in Preventive Medicine and Public Health by the American Board of Preventive Medicine and is also Board-Certified in Addiction Medicine by the American Board of Addiction Medicine.